EVALUATING OUTCOMES IN HEALTH AND SOCIAL CARE

Helen Dickinson and Janine O'Flynn

Second Edition

First edition published in Great Britain in 2008

This edition published in Great Britain in 2016 by

Policy Press
University of Bristol
1-9 Old Park Hill
Bristol BS8 1SD
UK
t: +44 (0)117 954 5940
pp-info@bristol.ac.uk
www.policypress.co.uk

North America office:
Policy Press
c/o The University of Chicago Press
1427 East 60th Street
Chicago, IL 60637, USA
t: +1 773 702 7700
f: +1 773 702 9756
sales@press.uchicago.edu
www.press.uchicago.edu

British Library Cataloguing in Publication Data
A catalogue record for this book is available from the British Library

Library of Congress Cataloging-in-Publication Data
A catalog record for this book has been requested

ISBN 978-1-4473-2976-3 paperback
ISBN 978-1-4473-2978-7 ePub
ISBN 978-1-4473-2977-0 Mobi

Cover design by Policy Press
Printed and bound in Great Britain by Lavenham Press Ltd, Suffolk
Policy Press uses environmentally responsible print partners

Contents

List of tables, figures and boxes

Tables

Figures

Boxes

Acknowledgements

Helen and Janine would like to acknowledge the contribution of a number of people who have allowed them to draw on and use their work in this book. Thanks go to Jon Glasby for allowing them to draw on his work with Helen Dickinson (Box 2.4) and to Helen Sullivan for allowing them to draw on her work with Helen Dickinson in Chapter 3; Asthana and colleagues for Figure 3.2; Emma Miller for allowing them to use Table 4.1; Woodland and Hutton for Figure 4.1; Jon Glasby, Stephen Jeffares, Helen Sullivan and Alison Nicholds for allowing them to reproduce Table 4.2; and Chris Ham and colleagues for allowing them to draw on their work (Box 4.3). Finally, thanks also go to George Cox for his assistance in the final stages of the book in terms of formatting and bringing together references.

Any personal opinions (or errors) in the book are those of the authors.

List of abbreviations

Health and social care use a large number of abbreviations and acronyms, and some of the more popular terms used in this book are set out below:

AEGIS	Aid to the Elderly in Government Institutions
ASCOT	Adult Social Care Outcomes Toolkit
CAT	Collaboration Assessment Tool
CCG	clinical commissioning group
CCT	compulsory competitive tendering
DALY	disability-adjusted life year
HoNOS 65+	Health of the Nation Outcome Scale for older people
HoNOSCA	Health of the Nation Outcome Scale for children and adolescents
LSP	local strategic partnership
NHS	National Health Service
NPM	new public management
ODPM	Office of the Deputy Prime Minister
OECD	Organisation for Economic Co-operation and Development
POET	Partnership Outcomes Evaluation Toolkit
QALY	quality-adjusted life year
RCT	randomised controlled trial
RDT	resource dependency theory
RE	realistic evaluation
SCIE	Social Care Institute for Excellence
ToC	theories of change

All web references in the following text were correct at the time of printing.

Preface

Whenever you talk to people using health and social services, they often assume that the different agencies and professions talk to each other regularly, actively share information and work closely together. Indeed, most people don't distinguish between 'health' and 'social care' at all – or between individual professions such as 'nursing', 'social work' or 'occupational therapy'. They simply have 'needs' that they want addressing in a professional and responsive manner – ideally by someone they know and trust. How the system is structured behind the scenes could not matter less.

And yet, people working in health and social care know that it *does* matter. None of us starts with a blank sheet of paper, and we all have to finds ways of working in a system that was not designed with integration in mind. As the books in this series explain, different parts of our health and social care services have evolved over time as largely separate entities, and policy-makers, managers and front-line practitioners trying to offer a joined-up service will typically face a series of practical, legal, financial and cultural barriers. This is often time-consuming and frustrating, and the end result for service users and their families often still does not feel very integrated (no matter how hard the professionals were working to try to produce a joint way forward). As one key commentator suggests, 'you can't integrate a square peg into a round hole' (Leutz, 1999, p 93).

When services aren't joined-up, it can result in poor outcomes for everybody – gaps, duplication and wasted time and resources. People using services frequently express amazement at the number of different people they have to tell their story to. Instinctively, it doesn't feel like a good use of their time or of the skilled professionals who are trying to help them. Often, one part of the system can't do something until they've had input from another part, and this can lead to all kinds of delays, inefficiencies and missed opportunities.

For staff, it can be surprisingly difficult to find enough time and space to gain a better understanding of how other agencies and professions operate, what they do, what priorities they have and what constraints they face. For someone who went into a caring profession to make a difference, there is nothing more dispiriting than knowing that someone needs a joined-up response but not knowing how to achieve it. In many situations, workers feel they are being asked to help people with complex needs, but with one hand constantly tied behind their back.

For the broader system, this state of affairs seems equally counter-productive. If support is delayed or isn't sufficiently joined-up, it can lead to needs going unmet and to people's health rapidly deteriorating. It then becomes even harder and even more expensive to intervene in a crisis – and this leaves less time and money for other people who are becoming unwell and need support (thus creating a vicious cycle). Poor communication, duplication and arguments over who should pay for what all lead to inefficiency, bad feeling and poor outcomes for people using services. In extreme cases, a lack of joint working can also culminate in very serious, tragic situations – such as a child death, a mental health homicide, the abuse of a person with learning difficulties or an older person dying at home alone (see Box 0.1 for but one high profile example). Here, partnership working is quite literally a matter of life and death, and failure to collaborate can have the most serious consequences for all involved.

Box 0.1: Partnership working as a matter of life or death

Following the tragic death of Peter Connelly (initially known as 'Baby P' in the press), Lord Laming (2009) was asked to produce a national review of progress since his initial investigation into the equally horrific death of Victoria Climbié in the same borough of Haringey (Laming, 2003). As the 2009 review observed (Laming, 2009, para 4.3):

> It is evident that the challenges of working across organisational boundaries continue to pose barriers in practice, and that cooperative efforts are often the first to suffer when services and individuals are under pressure. Examples of poor practice highlighted to this report include child protection conferences where not all the services involved in a child's life are present or able to give a view; or where one professional disagrees with a decision and their view is not explored in more detail; and repeated examples of professionals not receiving feedback on referrals. As a result of each of these failures, children or young people at risk of neglect or abuse will be exposed to greater danger. The referring professional may also be left with ongoing anxiety and concern about the child or young person. This needs to be addressed if all local services are to be effective in keeping children and young people safe.

For health and social care practitioners, if you are to make a positive and practical difference to service users and patients, most of the issues you face will involve working with other professions and other organisations. For public service managers, partnership working is likely to occupy an increasing amount of your time and budget, and arguably requires different skills and approaches to those prioritised in traditional single agency training and development courses. For social policy students and policy-makers, many of the issues you study and/ or try to resolve inevitably involve multiple professions and multiple organisations. Put simply, people do not live their lives according to the categories we create in our welfare services – real-life problems are nearly always messier, more complex, harder to define and more difficult to resolve than this.

Policy context

In response, national and local policy increasingly calls for enhanced and more effective partnership working as a potential solution (see, for example, DH, 2013). While such calls for more joint working can be inconsistent, grudgingly made and/or overly aspirational, the fact remains that collaboration between different professions and different organisations is increasingly seen as the norm (rather than as an exception to the rule). This is exemplified in a previous Welsh policy paper, *The sustainable social services for Wales: A framework for action* (Welsh Assembly Government, 2011, p 11) that argued, 'We want to change the question from "how might we cooperate across boundaries?" to justifying why we are not.' With most new funding and most new policy initiatives, there is usually a requirement that local agencies work together to bid for new resources or to deliver the required service, and various Acts of Parliament place statutory duties of partnership on a range of public bodies. As an example of the growing importance of partnership working, in 1999 the word 'partnership' was recorded 6,197 times in official parliamentary records, compared to just 38 times in 1989 (Jupp, 2000, p 7). When we repeated this exercise for the first edition of this book, we found 17,912 parliamentary references to 'partnership' in 2006 alone (although this fell to 11,319 when removing references to legislation on civil partnerships that was being debated at the time). Since then, there have been two general elections/ new governments and a series of major spending cuts and pressures – arguably making joint working harder to achieve in practice, but even more important.

In 1998, the Department of Health issued a consultation document on future relationships between health and social care. Entitled *Partnership in action*, the document proposed various ways of promoting more effective partnerships, basing these on a scathing but extremely accurate critique of single agency ways of working:

> All too often when people have complex needs spanning both health and social care good quality services are sacrificed for sterile arguments about boundaries. When this happens people, often the most vulnerable in our society ... and those who care for them find themselves in the no man's land between health and social services. This is not what people want or need. It places the needs of the organisation above the needs of the people they are there to serve. It is poor organisation, poor practice, poor use of taxpayers' money – it is unacceptable. (DH, 1998, p 30)

Whatever you might think about subsequent policy and practice, the fact that a government document sets out such a strongly worded statement of its beliefs and guiding principles is important. How to move from the rhetoric to reality is always the key challenge – but such quotes illustrate that partnership working is no longer an option (if it ever was), but core business. Under the coalition government (2010-15), this previous language shifted once again – and most recent policy refers to the importance of 'integrated care' (rather than 'partnerships' or 'collaboration'). As the coalition's NHS Future Forum (2012, p 3) argued:

> Integration is a vitally important aspect of the experience of health and social care for millions of people. It has perhaps the greatest relevance for the most vulnerable and those with the most complex and long-term needs. We have services to be proud of, and patients in England already receive some of the most joined-up services in the world. However, too many people fall through gaps between services as they traverse journeys of care which are often too difficult for them to navigate themselves. This lack of integration results daily in delays and duplication, wasted opportunities and

patient harm. It is time to "mind the gaps" and improve the experience and outcomes of care for people using our services.

While it is not always fully clear what a commitment to more integrated care might mean in practice (see below for further discussion), recent policy seems to be trying to achieve a number of different things, including:

- greater *vertical integration* between acute, community and primary care
- greater *horizontal integration* between community health and social care
- more effective joint working between *public health* and local government
- more effective partnerships between the *public, private and voluntary sectors*
- more *person-centred care*, with services that feel integrated to the patient.

In response to all this, the time feels right for a second edition of this book and of our 'Better partnership working' Series more generally. While our overall approach remains the same (see below for a summary of our aims and ethos), key changes to this edition include:

- updated references to current policy and practice
- the addition of more recent studies and broader literature
- a greater focus on 'integrated care' under the coalition government (2010-15) and the Conservative government of 2015-
- new reflective exercises and updated further reading/resources
- updated 'hot topics' (with a particular focus in some of the books in the series on the importance of working together during a time of austerity).

Aims and ethos

Against this background, this book (and the overall series of which it is part) provides an introduction to partnership working via a series of accessible 'how to' resources (see Box 0.2). Designed to be short and easy to use, they are nevertheless evidence-based and theoretically robust. A key aim is to provide *rigour and relevance* via books that:

- offer practical support to those working with other agencies and professions and to provide some helpful frameworks with which to make sense of the complexity that partnership working entails;
- summarise current policy and research in a detailed but accessible manner;
- provide practical but also evidence-based recommendations for policy and practice.

Box 0.2: The series at a glance

- *Partnership working in health and social care* (Jon Glasby and Helen Dickinson, 2nd edn)
- *Managing and leading in inter-agency settings* (Helen Dickinson and Gemma Carey, 2nd edn)
- *Interprofessional education and training* (John Carpenter and Helen Dickinson, 2nd edn)
- *Working in teams* (Kim Jelphs, Helen Dickinson and Robin Miller, 2nd edn)
- *Evaluating outcomes in health and social care* (Helen Dickinson and Janine O'Flynn, 2nd edn)

While each book is cross-referenced with others in the series, each is a standalone text with all you need to know as a student, practitioner, manager or policy-maker to make sense of the difficulties inherent in partnership working. In particular, the series aims to provide some practical examples to illustrate the more theoretical knowledge of social policy students, and some theoretical material to help make sense of the practical experiences and frustrations of front-line workers and managers.

Although there is a substantial literature on partnership working (see, for example, Hudson, 2000; Payne, 2000; Rummery and Glendinning, 2000; Balloch and Taylor, 2001; 6 et al, 2002; Glendinning et al, 2002; Sullivan and Skelcher, 2002; Barrett et al, 2005; Glasby and Dickinson, 2014, for just some of many potential examples), most current books are either broad edited collections, very theoretical books that are inaccessible for students and practitioners, or texts focusing on partnership working for specific user groups. Where more practical, accessible and general texts exist, they typically lack any real depth or evidence base – in many ways, they are little more than partnership 'cookbooks' that give apparently simple instructions that are meant to lead to the perfect and desired outcome. In practice, anyone who has studied or worked in health and social care knows that partnership working can be both frustrating and messy – even if you follow the so-called 'rules', the end result is often hard to predict, ambiguous and likely to provoke different reactions from different agencies and professions. In contrast, this book series seeks to offer a more 'warts and all' approach to the topic, acknowledging the realities that practitioners, managers and policy-makers face in the real world.

Wherever possible, the series focuses on key concepts, themes and frameworks rather than on the specifics of current policy and organisational structures (which inevitably change frequently). As a result, the series will hopefully be of use to readers in all four countries of the UK as well as other national settings. That said, where structures and key policies have to be mentioned, they will typically be those in place in England.

While the focus of the series is on public sector health and social care, it is important to note from the outset that current policy and practice also emphasises a range of additional partnerships and relationships, including:

- broader partnerships (for example, with services such as transport and leisure in adult services and with education and youth justice in children's services);
- collaboration not just between services, but also between professionals and people who use services;
- relationships between the public, private and voluntary sectors.

As a result, many of the frameworks and concepts in each book may focus initially on public sector health and social care, but will also be relevant to a broader range of practitioners, students, services and service users.

Ultimately, the current emphasis on partnership working and on integration means that everything about public services – their organisation and culture, professional education and training, inspection and quality assurance – will have to change. Against this background, we hope that this series of books is a contribution, however small, to these changes.

Jon Glasby and Helen Dickinson
University of Birmingham and University of Melbourne
December 2015

1

What are evaluation and outcomes, and why do they matter?

Evaluation is often considered to be a rather specialist and technical term, but we all engage in evaluation activities on a daily basis. At its most basic level evaluation may be considered the 'process of determining the merit, worth or value of something, or the product of that process' (Scriven, 1991, p 139). In deciding what car or cornflakes to buy we are making a comparative judgement about the worth or merit of the different cars or cornflakes available based on the information we have access to. Usually we are looking to get best value for the money we spend, or to find the product or service that is most suited to our needs and tastes.

We don't only make judgements over the worth or merit of products and services that we are personally involved with purchasing, however. Whether it is reports of taxpayers' money being 'wasted' through private-financed hospitals, large-scale procurements of computer systems for various public services, or re-branding services such as the Highways Agency, not a day goes by when there is not some report in the media over the alleged misuse of tax-funded services, organisations or products. The TaxPayers' Alliance (2014) goes as far as to estimate that £120 billion of taxpayers' money in the UK is 'wasted' annually – at least in terms of their evaluation. In a context of austerity and dramatic reductions to public spending budgets, if correct, this is a significant amount of money. Yet such conclusions are derived on the basis of a series of judgements and assumptions about the way the world is and should be. Typically, we do not evaluate tax-funded services simply to make sure that they are providing value for money on a cost basis. We also want to make sure that individuals using these services receive high quality services and products. Although choice holds a prominent place in the healthcare agenda (at least rhetorically), realistically, many of us in the past have typically had little choice over from whom or where we receive public services, and would expect all public services to offer the same high standards. Moreover, individuals with complex or chronic conditions may not be able to either actively judge the quality of services they receive, or have little to compare it to. Such services need to be evaluated to ensure that individuals have access to quality services that they want and need. Therefore it is essential that we systematically assess services, and ensure that public services are effective, efficient and delivered in line with the preferences and needs of users.

Collaborative working has assumed a prominent position within public policy not only in the UK but also more widely throughout the developed world. Writing from an Australian perspective, O'Flynn (2009, p 112) argues that 'a cult of collaboration' has emerged as this concept has become '*du jour* in Australian policy circles.' Similar sorts of arguments have been made in the US, continental Europe and a range of other jurisdictions (Haynes, 2015). Often the rhetoric driving the enthusiasm for collaboration relates to the provision of better services for those who use them, and an aspiration to 'create joined-up solutions to joined-up problems'. This argument has been further supported by a series of high-profile cases (some of which were indicated in Box 0.1) where the inability to work effectively in partnership has been presented as a major source of failure, which can have very real, negative consequences for individuals.

As McCray and Ward (2003) and others have suggested, collaboration often appears as a 'self-evident truth', yet it has still not been unequivocally demonstrated that working jointly improves outcomes for individuals who use public services. Despite the huge amount of time and money that has gone into working collaboratively in health and social care and evaluating the resultant impact, there is still a distinct lack of empirical evidence, particularly in terms of service user outcomes. This might be considered problematic in itself (given that collaborative working has assumed a central role in many areas of public policy), but in a context where governments across the UK have argued for the importance of evidence-based policy and practice, it might be considered even more remiss. Evaluation of the outcomes of collaborative working therefore remains an imperative, if not overdue, task. Yet, as we will see during the course of this text, this is often far from an easy process. This book is the revised edition of the original text. In the eight years since initial publication, the literatures on evaluation and collaboration have grown substantially, and yet many of the questions that were unanswered in the earlier edition remain so today. There have, however, been some significant steps forward in terms of the degree to which outcomes are understood and accepted as important measures across the fields of health and social care, and also in terms of the sophistication of evaluation approaches. Although we still lack definitive data concerning the impacts of collaborative working, a patchwork of evidence is emerging that fills in some of these gaps.

This edition has been updated in terms of the policy context and the evidence nationally and internationally, as well as receiving a complete overhaul in terms of hot topics and emerging issues, frameworks and tools. Our intention is that this should provide relevant up-to-date background information and the tools needed for individuals and teams seeking to evaluate outcomes in collaborative settings.

This chapter explores the health and social care literature to provide practical definitions of key terms in order to help readers think through the types of impacts that health and social care organisations may have for those who use their services and the ways in which we might evaluate this. One of the challenges in this field is that much of the language of evaluation and impact will likely be familiar to most of us and is in common use across many activities in our lives. While this familiarity is in some senses helpful, it can also be limiting, as when used in a context of systematic and scientific evaluation, meanings are typically more specific than everyday usage affords.

The chapter summarises the evolution of health and social care evaluation, and progressions within the field from an interest in inputs and outputs to more quality-based measures associated with outcomes.

We also provide an overview of the current political context and interest in evidence-based policy/practice and outcomes, and the associated implications these hold for performance management, accountability and inspection.

Evaluation

As already suggested, evaluation is a broad concept. Within the social sciences it has been described as a family of research methods which involves the:

> ... systematic application of social research procedures in assessing the conceptualisation and design, implementation, and utility of social intervention programs. In other words, evaluation research involves the use of social research methodologies to judge and to improve the planning, monitoring, effectiveness, and efficiency of health, education, welfare, and other human service programs. (Rossi and Freeman, 1985, p 19)

The systematic part of this definition is important because this tends to differentiate these evaluative approaches from the types of judgements that we make in our everyday lives (for example, about brands of cornflakes or what car to buy). In our everyday life we will typically draw on available information or may, with bigger or more considered decisions, seek out particular sources of data. The science of evaluation typically goes beyond this, considering what precisely is being evaluated, the information needed to do this, and carefully selects methods to collect and analyse information (Lazenbatt, 2002). Describing evaluation as a 'family of research methods' means that this activity may take many different forms, depending on the type of project and the aims of the evaluation. These varied approaches have often grown out of different academic disciplines or backgrounds and are underpinned by different sets of assumptions. An overview of some of the main types of evaluations that you may encounter within health and social care are set out in Box 1.1. Although presented here as separate types, in reality evaluation can incorporate several of these dimensions within the same project. Theory-led approaches (see Chapter 3), in particular, may be both formative and summative, evaluating process(es) and outcome(s). Some of these different types are more suited to particular stages of a programme to capture particular activities, and Box 1.1 provides an example of this (see also Figure 1.1).

Box 1.1: Common evaluation types used in health and social care

- *Feasibility evaluation* aims to appraise the possible effects of a programme before it has been implemented. That is, it aims to uncover all the possible consequences and costs of a particular proposed action before it has actually been implemented.
- *Process evaluation* typically looks at the 'processes' that go on within the service or programme that is being evaluated. Process evaluations normally help internal and external stakeholders to understand the way in which a programme operates, rather than what it produces.
- *Outcome or impact evaluation* assesses the outcomes or wider impacts of a programme against the programme's goals. An outcome evaluation may be a part of a summative evaluation (see below), but would not be part of a process evaluation.
- *Summative evaluation* tends to be used to help inform decision-makers to decide whether to continue a particular programme or policy. In essence, the aim of this type of research tends to concentrate on outputs and outcomes in order to 'sum up' or give an assessment of the effects and efficiency of a programme.
- *Formative evaluation* differs from summative evaluation in that it is more developmental in nature. It is used to give feedback to the individuals who are able to make changes to a programme so that it can be improved. Formative evaluations are interested in the processes that go on within a programme, but they also look at outcomes and outputs, and use this information to feed back into this process.

- *Implementation evaluation* assesses the degree to which a programme was implemented. Usually this involves being compared to a model of an intended programme, and analysing the degree to which it differs from its intended purposes.

- *Economic evaluation* aims to establish the efficiency of an intervention by looking at the relationship between costs and benefits. Not all the costs encountered within this approach are necessarily 'monetary'-based, and branches such as welfare economics consider 'opportunity costs' from a societal perspective (for further details, see Raftery, 1998).

- *Pluralistic evaluation* attempts to answer some of the critiques of outcome or impact evaluations that are thought to value some views of what constitutes success over others. Often evaluations take their referents of success from the most powerful stakeholders (often the funders of evaluations), which could potentially ignore other (perhaps more valid, in the case of service users?) perspectives. Pluralistic evaluation investigates the different views of what success is and the extent to which a programme was a success.

One explanation for why there are so many different types of evaluation approaches is that there is a range of different reasons why we evaluate. In thinking about measuring performance, Behn (2003) notes eight different reasons why we might wish to understand how teams or organisations are doing (see Box 1.2). These different reasons have implications in terms of the types of approaches we would likely adopt, and the data that would be needed to evaluate performance.

Figure 1.1: Focus of different types of evaluation

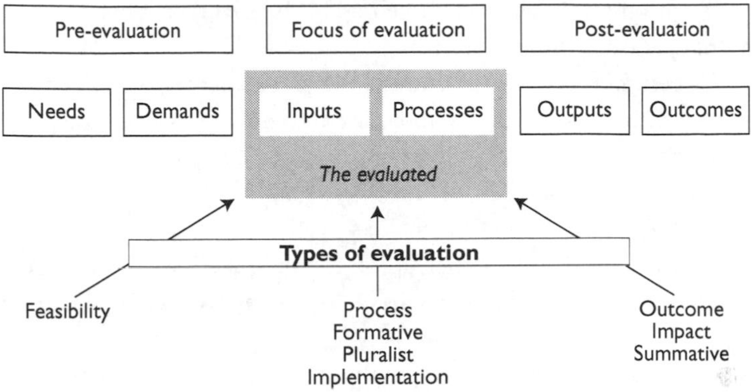

Source: Adapted from Øvretveit (1998, p 41)

Box 1.2: Eight reasons for measuring performance

- *Evaluate:* How well is my team or organisation performing?
- *Control:* How can I make sure my staff are doing the right thing?
- *Budget:* What should my organisation spend public money on?
- *Motivate:* How can I get staff, partners and citizens to do the right sorts of things to improve performance?
- *Promote:* How can I convince others that my team or organisation are doing a good job?
- *Celebrate:* Which things should we highlight as a success?
- *Learn:* What is and is not working?
- *Improve:* What should we change in order to improve how we perform?

Shadish and colleagues (1991) chart the history of evaluation theory, and note areas of disagreement between different evaluation types in terms of:

- the role of the evaluator;
- which values should be represented in the evaluation;
- the questions the evaluator should ask;
- the best methods (given limited time and resources);
- how the evaluator can try to ensure findings are used;
- which factors do or should influence the above choices about role, values, questions, methods and utilisation.

Despite these differences, they go on to note that there are four areas of agreement that tend to exist between different types of evaluations:

- evaluations are usually made within time and resource constraints that call for trade-offs;
- evaluators are rarely welcomed;
- there are limitations to any single evaluation;
- evaluators need to be more active in ensuring that their findings are acted on.

These observations paint a less than positive perspective of the field of evaluation and its practical implementation, but arguably hold true today as much as they did a quarter of a century ago when written. But what these do remind us is that there are no easy answers when it comes to evaluation; this can prove to be a difficult process characterised by tough decisions and trade-offs. For starters it is not always immediately apparent which is the best approach to take within a particular situation. Evaluation types range in the methods that they draw on. For example, many of the more process-led approaches have tended to incorporate qualitative approaches (for example, semi-structured or unstructured interviews, focus groups, ethnography) as their primary sources of data, while impact and outcome evaluations have often prioritised quantitative approaches (for example, experimental and quasi-experimental studies, structured interviews, questionnaires).

The debate over the benefits of qualitative versus quantitative approaches is rife throughout the evaluation and methodology literatures (see, for example, Kirk and Miller, 1986; Singleton et al,

1988). We do not intend to rehearse the detail of this debate in this book, as others have done so in much greater detail than we have the space to do here, and we point readers to some useful sources at the end of the chapter. It would also be disingenuous to say that this debate has been (or ever will be) settled or will ever reach an agreed outcome. While the more academic debates will continue, in practice many commentators would agree with us that that no method is intrinsically superior, and that more pragmatic approaches are needed when determining which approaches are more appropriate in particular contexts. Adopting this 'horses for courses' position (Silverman, 2013) means that it is important that you are clear about what you are aiming to evaluate and why, a point that is central in Behn's reasons to measure (see Box 1.2), and which we explore further in Chapter 3.

Having noted that it is important to know what you are evaluating, we now move to consider what kinds of things you might be interested in exploring.

Inputs, outputs and outcomes

As we describe below in the policy overview, outcomes have traditionally been overlooked in health and social care in favour of inputs and outputs. Today, although the political discourse has moved on to centrally incorporate considerations of outcomes, the practice often still tends to reflect a preference for inputs and outputs. It may seem like there is only a rather minor distinction between these terms (particularly in terms of outputs and outcomes), but these can have major implications for what those involved in service delivery focus attention on, what evaluators are able to talk about with confidence and even more importantly, for those who use services. Definitions of these terms are set out in Box 1.3, but it is also worth us elaborating on them with an example of evaluation in health and social care. If we wanted to understand the impact of an integrated team providing services to older people, we could measure the number of people who receive these services, and if we know that one of the aims of these services is to support people to live at home independently for longer, we might also be interested in understanding where service users live (for example, home/residential care). These would be relatively simple measures of outputs and might give us a limited understanding of the results of this team. What this would not tell us is whether the lives of these older people are good or bad relative to the norm. What we would miss by just focusing on output measures is whether this residential status is the most appropriate indicator, and that this is having the intended overall impact on the lives of these individuals. To obtain a sense of this we would need to incorporate some form of outcome measure (we consider examples of possible measures in more detail in Chapter 4).

Looking at a different policy field, the aspired outcome of employment services is often described as being an individual securing employment. However, according to the definitions in Box 1.3, we can see that this may be more correctly described as an output, as it tells us nothing about the impact of this job on the life of an individual or family. If this job has uncertain hours, is of poor quality, or some distance from home involving a long commute, it may lead to worse outcomes for an individual, and could even put pressure on other types of services. As the focus on outcomes has come to gain greater traction in recent years, we have seen a number of debates emerge as to whether particular factors are outputs or outcomes (see, for example, de Bruijn, 2002). Alongside this increasingly complex debate, most have tended to assume that inputs are far more certain and simple to measure. This may be the case for some inputs, but when we look closely at collaborative working, it might actually be quite difficult to sum up all the 'invisibles' that enable joined-up approaches (such as the time it takes in terms of meetings or building relationships between professionals) and to quantify this accurately. A key lesson here is that it is rarely clear which aspects of inputs, outputs and outcomes should be taken into consideration: the deciding of these factors is not always obvious, and often involves taking a decision appropriate to the specific context in which the evaluation is taking place and the purposes of that evaluation (again, we discuss this further later on, in Chapter 2).

Box 1.3: Distinction between inputs, outputs and outcomes

Inputs are the resources (human, material or financial) that are used to carry out activities and produce outputs and/or accomplish results, for example, social workers, teachers, books, computers, beds, medical instruments. *Outputs* refer to the effects of a process (such as a service) on an administrative structure (Axford and Berry, 2005). They are the direct products or services that stem from the activities of initiatives, and are delivered to a specific group or population, for example, maternal healthcare service visits, medical procedures undertaken. *Outcomes* are the 'impact, effect or consequence of help received' (Nicholas et al, 2003, p 2). That is, outcomes are not just the direct products or services, but are the totality of the consequences of the actions of an organisation, policy, programme or initiative. In other words, outcomes are the 'impact on society of a particular public sector activity' (Smith, 1996, p 1), for example, child wellbeing, social inclusion, community safety.

If the distinction between outputs and outcomes is not enough of a challenge, there is a further dimension to definitions of outcomes. As Box 1.4 illustrates, outcomes may be further differentiated into at least three forms: service process, change and maintenance outcomes. Service process outcomes have increasingly been demonstrated to play a substantial role in the difference that services make in terms of their overall effect. Many of us will have at some time received or purchased services from someone who seemed genuinely interested and made sure you received the highest quality services. Where this happens you are not only more likely to go back there again, but are also more likely to follow any advice the service provider might give, be more willing to offer information, and generally feel more positive and engaged with that situation than if you feel like you are a burden on that professional or service. An important message for service providers is that, to some degree, 'it ain't what you do, it's the way you do it'. This is a particularly important message for those involved in the delivery of services in the sense that these are always co-produced between the deliverer and the receiver. Co-produced services cannot be quality controlled prior to delivery, and each action of delivery is unique (Alford, 2009). To this extent services are intangible (they can't be stored or tested in advance), heterogeneous (individuals will have different priorities) and inseparable (they can't be produced without interacting with service users) (Lewis and Hartley, 2001).

In the past, service process outcomes have often been overlooked in some areas of public services. To some degree this is due to the hangover of the attitude that individuals should be grateful to receive any services, let alone the ones they want, and where and when they want them. However, it has begun to be recognised, both in research and by central government (to an extent), just how important this factor is in the delivery of services (more of which in Chapter 3). Indeed, it may be that how services are received not only has an impact on the output but also the end outcome that we are seeking – the means matter, and understanding these processes is important to evaluating services.

Box 1.4: Different forms of outcomes

Service process outcomes reflect the impact of the way in which services are delivered. This might include the degree to which service users are treated as human beings; feel that their privacy and confidentiality are respected; or treated as people with the right to services.

Change outcomes are improvements made in physical, mental or emotional functioning. This includes improvements in symptoms of depression or anxiety that impair relationships and impede social participation, in physical functioning and in confidence and morale (Qureshi et al, 1998).

Maintenance outcomes are those that prevent or delay deterioration in health, wellbeing or quality of life. This can include low-level interventions and their outcomes such as living in a clean and tidy environment and having social contact.

Just as the professions and procedures of health and social care have developed separately (see Glasby and Dickinson, 2014, for further discussion), so, too, have their outcome indicators. Consequently, conceptualisations of 'medical' and 'social' outcomes and the ways in which we measure these are often quite different in practice. Social care outcomes are traditionally wider in perspective and concerned with everyday aspects of life; medical indicators are predominantly allied with 'negative' (that is, disease-free) views of health and tend to be associated with clinical indicators embedded in the quantitative approach (Young and Chesson, 2006). Typically what this means is that social care outcomes can be more difficult to measure than medical outcomes, although precise measurement may be less of an issue in this context when social care is often more concerned with maintenance than change outcomes. The majority of social care is about maintaining a level, or preventing further deterioration, rather than making specific improvements in users' lives. Qureshi et al (1998) estimate that around 85% of social care work is directed at sustaining an acceptable quality of life. The difference between services aiming to achieve change and services aspiring to continually maintain levels of outcome has clear implications for the ways they are assessed and interpreted. Research investigating the impact of collaborative working often has to find a way to bring together different forms and measures of success, which can be a challenging process given the different starting assumptions of approaches.

Without wishing to add even further complexity, there is one more dimension that we need to consider in gaining a full perspective on outcomes: timescales. One of the challenges in measuring outcomes is that they are not always immediately obvious and it can take an extended period of time to fully understand the implications of a set of activities. The beauty of outputs is that they are often more apparent, which means that they are often more compatible with political timescales than outcomes (and we illustrate this with examples later on in the book). To deal with this challenge we can break down outcomes into what these might look like in terms of immediate, intermediate and long-term outcomes (see Figure 1.2).

Figure 1.2: Immediate, intermediate and end outcomes

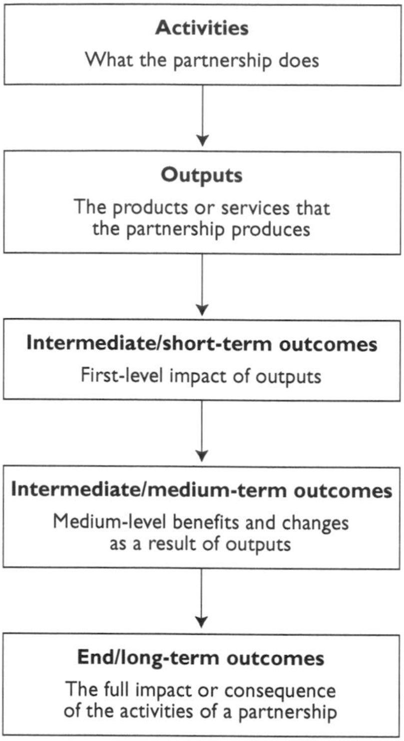

While a helpful way to think about outcomes, we have to contend with the fact that inter-agency collaborations often centre round complex (or 'wicked') issues, and this might mean that outcomes operate at multiple levels and have an impact on stakeholders in different ways. What looks like a good outcome for one group might not be quite as positive for another, and different organisations will likely have varying views on outcomes and timescales. Although it may be the case that collaboration can improve the user experience, it could lead to professionals feeling overwhelmed as a result of increased workload (Bruner, 1991) or 'partnership fatigue' from attending many meetings for different collaborative initiatives (Huxham and Vangen, 2004). Depending on what we are trying to evaluate, we might want to examine a range of types of outcomes manifest at different times and for multiple stakeholder groups, or simply focus on one particular aspect of a service. More holistic evaluation approaches may provide a very different assessment of our activity.

Policy overview

Over the past 30 years we have seen a rapid expansion in the industry of performance management, and as a consequence the interest and investment made in processes of evaluation. Traditionally, public services relied on systems of informal peer scrutiny, with professionals responsible for ensuring their colleagues were operating in a moral and ethical manner. There was an implicit compact, particularly in healthcare, whereby professionals largely operated autonomously in return for being self-regulating. However, these systems were often considered opaque and closed to all but a special few groups (Harrison, 1999).This tended to be a relatively simple way to measure the activity and performance of health and social care services that was not overly expensive and did not require extra analysis by external evaluators. But such approaches were considered unacceptable to many, and a number of separate movements and activities have conspired, over time, to change this to a situation where performance management is both more formalised and transparent, and the actions and activities of these actors are more open to scrutiny. We reflect here on these different drivers and the emphasis that they have, in turn, called for in evaluations of performance in health and care services. Although we focus on the UK context, the major themes have been observed across many other developed countries, with a slightly different emphasis, over the past quarter century or so.

The first driver we consider is the voice of service users. Ham (1977) describes that in the 1960s organisations representing patients became a more important and challenging force for government in the UK. Examples of such organisations include the Patients' Association, the

National Association of Mental Health and the National Association for the Welfare of Children in Hospital, among others. These organisations highlighted the fact that services were not always of the quality or order that service users expected, and not all professionals were operating on the basis of best practice or patient interest. The government responded to this by gradually trying to incorporate a stronger voice into the NHS through community health councils and other subsequent initiatives.

These actions were strengthened by emerging evidence that care standards more broadly were not necessarily keeping pace with community expectations. Barbara Robb and the pressure group AEGIS (Aid to the Elderly in Government Institutions) highlighted low standards of care for older people in British hospitals. Robb (1967) published a collection of essays and articles that revealed a disturbing indictment of seven hospitals where doctors, nurses and patients revealed conditions of neglect and incidents of ill treatment and brutality. These conditions were suggested to be the outcome of overcrowding, frayed nerves and even despair. This evidence was further supported by official inquiries such as that into conditions at Ely Hospital in Cardiff (DH, 1969), an institution for people with learning difficulties. The findings were widely publicised in the media and made the public aware of the nature of conditions that some of the UK's most vulnerable groups were encountering, which in turn put increasing pressure on government (for further discussion of the impact that a number of scandals have had on UK public services, see Butler and Drakeford, 2005).

A second factor that has been important in driving greater interest in performance measurement came through shifts in how the mainstream literature thinks about public management. In 1995, the Organisation for Economic Co-operation and Development (OECD) observed that 'a new paradigm for public management has emerged, aimed at fostering a performance-oriented culture in a less centralized public sector' (1995, p 8). New public management (NPM), although broadly recognisable internationally, varies from country to country in its implementation. It is essentially founded on a critique of bureaucracy as the organising principle of public administration (Dunleavy, 1991), considering it inflexible and overly hierarchical. Such a perspective argues that the top-down decision-making processes associated with bureaucracy are increasingly distant from the expectations of citizens. NPM theorists drew on the commercial sector for lessons, arguing that because of the large-scale international competition private sector organisations had been exposed to from the 1980s onwards, those that were successful had become increasingly efficient, while also offering consumers products that they wanted. The commercial sector had undergone radical change but it was argued that the public sector remained 'rigid and bureaucratic, expensive, and inefficient' (Pierre and Peters, 2000, p 5).

The principles of NPM are, in general, characterised as an approach that emphasises output controls; disaggregates traditional bureaucratic organisations and decentralises management authority; introduces market and quasi-market mechanisms; and strives for customer-oriented services. This way of working puts more emphasis on the importance of performance-managing outcomes, determining what it is that service users want from their health and social care services, and delivering this through flatter and less hierarchical structures. As Hood (1991) describes, these reforms are characterised by an increased decentralisation of power to local levels, with managers increasingly taking responsibility for budgets and being allowed greater flexibilities in terms of their actions, but simultaneously bearing more responsibility for the outputs and outcomes of that particular unit (see Dickinson and Carey, 2016, for further discussion of NPM).

Interest in NPM first came about in the late 1970s and early 1980s at a time when the UK was experiencing significant economic problems (for example, high rates of unemployment and inflation), in addition to long-standing criticisms over the quality of public services and their efficiency. One of the consequences of these reforms was the increased use of private firms and semi-government bodies to deliver services alongside traditional government bodies. For example, local government had to undertake compulsory competitive tendering (CCT) of goods and services where local authority-conducted work was compared against private sector provision. In local authorities, CCT increased the use of the private sector in providing public services, which in turn put more competitive pressure on the public sector. Since the time of CCT there has been an increasing trend for local authorities to purchase services from private and community sector organisations. Although this pattern has taken longer to establish in the healthcare sector (despite the fact that GPs have largely remained independent contractors throughout the history of the NHS), there has been a greater acceleration of this within the English NHS over the past decade (Greener, 2015). The NPM focus on efficiency and customer service has driven a major emphasis on performance and evaluation, the effects of which have been mixed. Pressures to change performance management systems, which have influenced a greater interest in the outcomes of health and social care services, have, over time, come from a variety of sources, including:

- pressure groups and calls for greater public voice in the delivery of health and social care services;
- a series of inquiries revealing inadequate conditions within a range of health and social care services (but primarily for vulnerable groups);
- the influence of NPM;
- increased division between providers and commissioners of public services;
- recognition that many of the 'wicked' issues that society faces cannot be solved by any one government agency or department operating independently, and that the actions of different departments have an impact on others, for example, increased recognition that a number of health issues have social, economic and political determinants, as well as biological.

As a result of these various factors, successive governments have been more concerned with outcomes (even if this is, at times, somewhat of a rhetorical interest). This was manifest under the New Labour governments of 1997-2010, most explicitly through the policy documents *Every Child Matters* (HM Treasury, 2003) that set out a list of outcomes that children's services should be aiming to achieve, and a joint health and social care White Paper, *Our health, our care, our say* (DH, 2006), which set out outcomes for adult services. Since 2010 the NHS Outcomes Framework has been used to set out annual national outcome goals that the Secretary of State uses to monitor the progress of NHS England. The NHS Outcomes Framework sits alongside the Adult Social Care and Public Health Outcomes Frameworks. The NHS Outcomes Framework is a set of 68 indicators that measure performance in the health and care system across five domains, as set out in Box 1.5.

Box 1.5: The five domains of the NHS Outcomes Framework

- Domain 1: Preventing people from dying prematurely
- Domain 2: Enhancing quality of life for people with long-term conditions
- Domain 3: Helping people recover from episodes of ill health or following injury
- Domain 4: Ensuring that people have a positive experience of care
- Domain 5: Treating and caring for people in a safe environment and protecting them from avoidable harm

---

As we can see from the brief summary of the policy context outlined here, performance management processes and an interest in outcomes have moved from being largely professionally dominated and opaque to all but a chosen few to being a central activity of professionals, firmly under the purview of government. This shift has occurred as the result of a number of diverse drivers that have come together to increase attention and interest in evaluation and outcomes. Today, the measurement of outcomes on a regular basis is an important activity of all health and social care organisations. In the next section we turn to consider the link between evidence and collaboration in health and social care.

Towards evidence-based health and social care collaboration?

One important issue that we did not cover in the discussion of the policy context set out above relates to the evidence-based movement. Over a similar sort of time frame that we have seen growing interest in performance management and outcomes there has been a rise in the interest afforded to evidence-based policy and practice. The evidence-based movement originally emerged from the field of medicine, but has since spread across public services nationally and internationally. The first New Labour government expressed a desire to be a thoroughly modernising force, and evidence was an important part of this process (Dickinson, 2014). The refrain 'what counts is what works' became somewhat of a mantra for this government, and since this time the importance of evidence in policy processes and the practice of public services has remained an important feature.

This trend has not just been confined to the UK, but is a theme throughout a range of different jurisdictions (Head, 2014). In Australia, former Prime Minister Kevin Rudd observed that 'evidence-based policy making is at the heart of being a reformist government' (quoted in Banks, 2009, p 3), and this was a sentiment shared across many other systems of government. In pursuit of resolving 'wicked' issues it is argued that the use of evidence across a range of partners is of particular importance (Head and O'Flynn, 2015).

The evidence-based movement is based on 'the conscientious, explicit, and judicious use of current best evidence in making decisions about the care of individual patients ... [which] means integrating individual ... expertise with the best available external ... evidence from systematic research' (Sackett et al, 1996, p 71). Gray (1997) argues that an enthusiasm for evidence-based policy and practice represents a shift away from making decisions simply on the basis of opinion. This is a powerful rhetorical point, although it would be an oversimplification and misrepresentation to suggest that prior to the evidence-based movement decisions were based on little more than opinions. What this turn does represent is an explicit move towards decision-making based on data that has been gathered and appraised according to sound principles of scientific enquiry.

While it seems that this is a reasonable premise from which to make vital policy decisions, the evidence-based movement is not without its critics. There are important debates over what constitutes 'valid' evidence, and which experts might hold this evidence (see, for example, Glasby and Beresford, 2006). Further, it is often argued that very specific types of evidence (for example, 'objective', quantitative data) are more scientific than others.

Aside from the challenges inherent in deciding which kinds of evidence are most valid or relevant within particular contexts, other commentators have also expressed less than favourable and occasionally cynical views of the evidence-based movement. Klein (2000), for example, suggests that a focus on evidence-based policy is a way of sheltering politicians from making difficult or unpopular decisions. When having to choose a particular course of action over another, they can do so by recourse to 'scientific evidence', when, in fact, the course of action may be more complex and politically motivated than this suggests. Interestingly, there is an equally passionate argument about how politicians ignore evidence in deciding policy directions and instead make 'political' rather than 'rational' decisions. The debate about the criminalisation and banning of a range of drugs is an excellent case in point – health experts have made the case against banning based on evidence, while some politicians ignore this for political, ideological or moral reasons (see Dunt, 2015, for a good discussion).

Regardless of the critics of the evidence-based movement, over the past 20 years we have seen a significant growth in the enthusiasm for, and investment in, evaluation in the context of public policy and public services. Although the UK has seen somewhat of a slow-down in investments in large-scale evaluations such as those of Health Action Zones and local strategic partnerships (LSPs), arguably evaluation processes have become a more central component of local organisational practice. Given the enthusiasm of successive governments for the use of evidence in decision-making practices and processes and for the pursuit of collaboration as the *modus operandi* of contemporary government, we might be excused for assuming that there is clear-cut evidence that working collaboratively across health and social care produces better outcomes for those accessing services. Yet, when we analyse the evidence, we find that evidence of performance improvement 'remains uncertain at best' (Dickinson and Sullivan, 2014, p 163). As we will see in the following chapter, there is some evidence pertaining to specific case studies and to some care groups, but we lack clear and consistent evidence to demonstrate that collaboration leads to better outcomes for those who use services despite this seeming a self-evident link.

If collaboration is as central to 21st-century government as the literature would suggest, and significant time and effort has been expounded in the pursuit of this agenda in a context of espoused preference for evidence-based policy, then it would seem remiss that we lack evidence to demonstrate these causal links. For some, this has resulted in a 'faith-based' rather than 'evidence-based' approach to collaboration (O'Flynn, 2009). For others, however, this is less of a problem than it might be assumed to be. In a report from the Public Policy Institute for Wales, Entwistle (2014, p 9) argues:

> In truth ... the balance of evidence is of less significance than it might first appear. Governments are faced by pressing social problems, diminishing resources and exponentially expanding complexity. It is increasingly self-evident that no single organisation can be expected to solve these problems acting alone. At the same time, it is impossible to conceive of an organisational re-design that would negate the need for cross boundary working. The problems facing contemporary societies cannot be resolved through improved hierarchical processes or free market competition. In the absence of alternative solutions to the challenges facing us, some form of partnership working – both between local authorities and a range of other agencies – appears to be the only game in town. Partnership working is then both an inevitable and desirable fact of contemporary public management.

What this quote illustrates so well is one of the central challenges of outcomes and collaboration. Such is the enthusiasm for the collaboration agenda that in the face of a lack of evidence of the impact of collaboration in terms of service user (or other) outcomes, it still appears to many that collaboration is the 'common sense' (Mason et al, 2015, p 178) response to a multiplicity of challenges that governments face. One of the dangers here is that we run the risk of treating collaboration as an end in itself, rather than as a means to an end, and we may overinvest in collaborative processes and practices. Without evaluating the outcomes of collaborative endeavours, we are assuming that they have the intended result and are treating these as an end (and not a means to an end). Over the longer term one of the potential risks of this situation is that the legitimacy of the collaborative endeavour may be undermined. After all, one thing that is well evidenced in the literature is the difficulty of collaborative working (Mitchell et al, 2015). If professionals experience collaborative working as a challenge on a day-to-day basis, and after nearly 20 years of the vigorous pursuit of this agenda within a context of (at least rhetorically) evidence-based policy and practice when we still lack evidence around this concept, then there is potential for this to erode enthusiasm in collaborative practice.

As Glasby and Dickinson (2014) point out, even over recent history there have been some profound changes in terms of the language we use to speak about this agenda. When the first editions of this series were written, the terminology was very much located around a partnership approach, although in recent years, with different governments and politics, this has shifted to integration. At its core are fundamentally the same sorts of ideas, but they have been labelled differently in order to continue to gain buy in. If anything, the key message of the books in this series is that making collaboration work is difficult and takes continual investment, time and intention. There is no one way to do collaboration, and approaches need to be appropriate to that locality. If professionals are not willing to engage with this agenda, then, put simply, collaboration will not happen.

We would therefore argue that it is important that we are able to effectively assess the outcomes of collaboration at a number of levels in order to be able to talk in a more evidence-informed way about the impacts of these mechanisms. This is an important exercise so that we know about the operation and impact of collaboration at a local and more collective level, but also in terms of the enthusiasm for collaboration as a political agenda. Having set out the background to these issues, the remainder of the book illustrates ways in which we can go about exploring the outcomes of collaboration in health and social care, what some of the major challenges are to this process and what the latest available data tells us about the processes and outcomes of collaborative working.

As indicated above, for some commentators a lack of evidence of the effectiveness of collaboration is not necessarily problematic. This may be in part because individuals have such a strong belief in this concept, but it is also due to the challenges in evaluating collaborative working. As Thomson et al (2009, p 29) conclude in their overview of the evaluation of collaboration literature, there are 'few instruments to measure collaboration ... and those that do are difficult to adapt outside the immediate context of a particular study.' The next chapter considers the scale of the challenge of evaluating collaboration in more detail, so we shall say little more of it here. Instead, this chapter concludes with Box 1.6, which gives an overview of the Sure Start programme that we use in this and the following two chapters to illustrate a number of the challenges of evaluating partnerships. While this real-life example is a few years old now, it represents one of the most complex, long-term (and expensive!) programmes of research into collaboration in the broader literature. We use this as a way of exemplifying many of the key issues in the book.

Box 1.6: An overview of Sure Start

Sure Start is an English government programme (with variants in Wales, Scotland and Northern Ireland) that aims to achieve better outcomes for children, parents and communities by:
- increasing the availability of childcare for all children;
- improving the health and emotional development of young children;
- supporting parents as parents, and in their aspirations towards employment.

When Sure Start was originally developed in 1998 it was hailed as a rather different programme to those that had previously been developed for children in England. Sure Start initiatives are area-based, focusing on all children and their families living in a prescribed area. The ultimate goal of these local Sure Start programmes was to enhance the life chances of children less than four years of age growing up in disadvantaged neighbourhoods. These local centres do not have a prescribed curriculum or set of services, but are charged with improving existing services and creating new ones as needed. In practice this has meant that quite varied approaches have been produced around the country, providing a diverse range of services. The expectation was that children in Sure Start areas would function and develop better than children who were yet to receive Sure Start services. In 2001 the National Evaluation of Sure Start was launched to test this assumption, and it ran to 2012. This evaluation was undertaken by a consortium of academics, but was led by Birkbeck College, University of London. In order to investigate the impacts of Sure Start, the team aimed to address three questions:

1. Have existing services changed?
2. Have delivered services been improved?
3. Have children, families and communities benefited?

For all three questions the research team also explored why any patterns of change existed, which groups experienced greatest impacts and under which conditions. There were five specific components to the evaluation (see Chapter 3 for further details), and it included a national survey of all the centres in addition to in-depth studies of 26. The evaluation team produced a series of reports outlining their findings over the course of the research process (see www.ness.bbk.ac.uk/).

The Head Start program in the US provides an interesting international comparison. With similar aims to Sure Start, it has been in operation since 1965, and many evaluations have been undertaken (see www.acf. hhs.gov/programs/ohs).

Reflective exercises

1. What does the term 'evaluation' mean to you, and why does it matter within health and social care settings?

2. Which of the different types of evaluation outlined in this chapter have you encountered? Are there any additional approaches that you know of that are not presented here? Compare and contrast your answer to this question with a colleague,

3. What do you understand by the terms 'inputs', 'outputs' and 'outcomes'? How do these factors differ from one another? How do they map onto a service that you have had involvement with?

4. Think about a collaboration you have either had personal experience of or read about. In what ways has it affected (positively or negatively) service outputs and service user outcomes? How do you know this? How could you go about formally measuring this?

5. Thinking about the Sure Start example outlined above, what do you think some of the key difficulties and complexities would be in evaluating the Sure Start programme? Which of the evaluation types outlined in this chapter do you think that the Sure Start evaluation should use? What might be some of the limitations and/or challenges of adopting such an approach?

Further reading and resources

- Relevant websites for official health and social care policy include:
  - Department of Health: www.dh.gov.uk
  - Department for Education: www.education.gov.uk
  - Department for Communities and Local Government: www. communities.gov.uk
- For general details on the Sure Start programme: www.nidirect.gov. uk/sure-start-services
- For information about the National Evaluation of Sure Start (including methodology and interim reports): www.ness.bbk.ac.uk/
- For an international comparison, visit the US Office of Head Start: www.acf.hhs.gov/programs/ohs
- For details on the debate between quantitative and qualitative approaches, the following sources are helpful:
  - Punch's (2014) *Introduction to social research*
  - Cresswell's (2014) *Research design*
- Key introductory textbooks on evaluation include:
  - Rossi and Freeman's (1985) *Evaluation*
  - Øvretveit's (1998) *Evaluating health interventions*
  - Nocon and Qureshi's (1996) *Outcomes of community care for users and carers*
  - Smith's (1996) *Measuring outcomes in the public sector*
- Sullivan's (2011) '"Truth" junkies: using evaluation in UK public policy' is a fascinating reflection on the experience of being involved in the evaluation of a number of prominent collaborative initiatives, and the status of evidence and its relationship to policy in the New Labour era.

2

What does research tell us?

In Chapter 1 we outlined the key contours of the discussions and debates around issues of outcomes and evaluation in health and social care, with particular reference to the challenges posed in the context of collaborative working. This chapter examines the evidence to draw lessons around issues such as the challenges in evaluating collaborative working; what the theoretical literature suggests collaboration should achieve; what collaboration has been demonstrated to achieve in practice; and the importance of clarity over drivers and outcomes. The key message of this chapter is that although individuals and groups often assume that collaboration is a common-sense response to a particular challenge or set of issues, the literature suggests that collaboration is driven by a variety of different imperatives. The lack of evidence of the link between collaborative practice and improved user outcomes may be partly due to the fact that individuals and groups are not always as clear as they might be in terms of what they are aiming to achieve through collaborative working. This lack of clarity can pose difficulties both in terms of achieving these aims in a practical sense, and being able to evidence these aspirations. Given this key message, it is perhaps fitting that we start by reflecting on the concept of collaboration, and what it is that is meant by it.

Challenge of 'collaboration'

Although collaboration seems like a relatively straightforward idea, it can be used to refer to a whole variety of different sorts of interactions. It generally denotes some sort of working relationship between two or more individuals or organisations, but beyond this there are a whole range of ways that these relationships may vary in terms of what links partners, why they are working together, how strong their bonds are, what form their relationship takes and to what ends. In a review of the evidence relating to the integration of funding in health and social care, Mason et al (2015) found at least eight different types of financial integration between parties (and we come back to these later in the chapter).

A number of commentators have suggested that the liberal use of collaboration (and allied terms) is problematic because it might lead to a loss of 'credibility, as it has become a catch-all for a wide range of concepts and a panacea for a multitude of ills. Partnerships can cover a wide spectrum of relationships and can operate at different levels, from informally taking account of other players, to having a constructive dialogue, working together on a project or service, joint commissioning and strategic alliances' (Banks, 2002, p 5). As far back as 1994, Leathard identified 52 separate terms being used to refer to collaboration, including interorganisational working, joint working, seamless working, joined-up thinking, interprofessional working, multiprofessional working, integrated teams, multiagency working, inter-agency working, collaboration and interdisciplinary working. She concludes, quite unsurprisingly, that the field is a 'terminological quagmire' (Leathard, 1994), and it is likely that this list of potential signifiers has only increased in the intervening years.

In evaluation terms this lack of specificity can pose somewhat of a challenge. In everyday life we are fairly used to deploying language in such a liberal way, and some (for example, McLaughlin, 2004) have argued that the very lack of definitional clarity has aided the popularisation of the concept. But for evaluators, this can be difficult. If we refer to lots of slightly different ways of working using the same word, it can make it difficult to talk with certainty about what the impact of particular processes or activities are. Further, different parties working together may have very different views on seemingly similar language, practices and activities.

As a result of this, a range of different frameworks or heuristics have been developed to aid researchers and evaluators to differentiate between different sorts of collaborative arrangements (see, for example, Hudson et al, 1999; Keast et al, 2007; Nolte and McKee, 2008; Curry and Ham, 2010). The challenge with many of these sorts of analytical tools is that they compare just one kind of thing. That is, they may compare number of partners, what links partners, the structure of relationships or reasons for working collaboratively. Yet collaborative arrangements might vary across a number of different dimensions, and by focusing on just one aspect by using a particular frame, we run the risk of assuming that this is the factor that has driven any impact and not others. Given the lack of precision on what we even mean by collaboration, it is not surprising that the jury is still out on whether joint working in health and social care actually improves outcomes. Some researchers find that collaboration 'works' (see, for example, Provan and Milward, 1995; Andrews and Entwistle, 2010), while others find either paucity of evidence or, in some cases, negative impacts. Within the broader literature on corporate alliances and partnerships, which covers corporate, community and public sector organisations, Hughes and Weiss (2007), for example, found that while the number of partnerships and alliances increased each year, the majority of these did not actually succeed. Similar findings are presented by Huxham and Vangen (2004), who argue that the likelihood of disappointing outcomes from collaborative endeavours is high.

The available evidence is not very convincing on the power of collaboration. A range of different studies find collaborative working has little impact in terms of improved outcomes for service users (Rummery, 2009; Hayes et al, 2011; Marek et al, 2014; Popp et al, 2014). And a systematic review examining the impact of inter-agency collaborations that target health outcomes and behaviours found that 'evidence of health benefit was extremely weak' (Hayes et al, 2011, p 19). The National Evaluation of the UK Department of Health's Integrated Care Pilots (RAND Europe and Ernst & Young, 2012, p 1) found that although staff believed improvements had been made, 'patients did not, in general, share the sense of improvement.' In addition, there was little evidence of a general reduction in emergency admissions, although there were some reductions in planned admissions and outpatient attendance. In their conclusions, the research team concur with the views of Powell Davies et al (2006), who argued that the most likely improvements following collaborative initiatives are in relation to healthcare processes and less likely to be apparent in terms of patient experience or reduced costs.

An interesting point emerges here: looking at collaboration from different viewpoints (patient, staff member, administrator, partner) may be very important in evaluating the importance, and impact, of joint working. Indeed, Huxham and Hibbert (2008) found in their work that there were five quite different views on success in collaborations: achieving outcomes; getting the processes to work; reaching emergent milestones; gaining recognition from others; and personal pride in championing a partnership. Deciding on what success would look like for a specific collaboration might not be quite so straightforward. In summary, the literature is fairly mixed. For some, collaboration seems to work, and for others, it does not, or we are at least less sure about whether it does or not. It is most often concluded that there is a differential impact across forms of arrangements and the client group being served. (We return to this issue in the next chapter, when we explore the different sorts of evidence we might wish to use to demonstrate impact in terms of different user groups.)

One final note worth making about the evidence base relating to collaborative working is that the focus of evaluations is still often on process, rather than service user outcomes. That is, they more often explore how effectively partners work together, rather than whether this makes any difference in terms of a range of different types of outcomes. There are many potential reasons for this state of affairs. One view of this might be that this is a reflection of the depth to which the assumption that partnerships inevitably lead to better outcomes is engrained within the public sector (and often evaluators' beliefs). If this is the case, rather than investigating service user outcomes, evaluators analyse the process of collaborative working, and if this seems smooth, presume that positive benefits must be being produced for service users. Process evaluations are cheaper and often far simpler to conduct, which is another reason for this trend. It requires significant investment and time to conduct an effective outcome evaluation and, as we will set out below in more detail, they are subject to a range of problems in terms of attribution. For this reason, Winkworth and Healy (2009, p 25) note that process evaluations of collaborations are generally viewed as a 'pragmatic, albeit second best solution.'

As noted in Chapter 1, even where lack of evidence concerning the efficacy of collaborative approaches is noted, commentators still often argue that either this is unproblematic (because there are no alternatives), or else evaluative challenges mean that we can't be definitive about the impacts of collaboration. In their study of integrated funding in health and social care, Mason et al (2015, p 186) find that:

> Only a small fraction of the schemes included in the review delivered significant improvements in health outcomes. This does not mean that policy makers should disregard the potential of integrated finance....The literature reveals that incomplete information ... was a common problem, and that even if cultural and governance differences were resolved at management level, budget holders might remain unable to provide their clients with access to appropriate services.

Collaboration and evaluation challenges

The impact of collaborative working is, therefore, uncertain, but what we do know from the literature is that collaboration is difficult to evaluate – and particularly so when we wish to increase the focus on outcomes rather than inputs, processes or outputs. Although we have briefly alluded to some of the factors already, we summarise these more fully in this section. We believe that it is important to do so as a reference for those who are embarking on the evaluation of collaborative endeavours (summarised in Box 2.1). Many of these issues are taxing indeed, and overcoming them will require substantial investment and/or time and effort. This is not to say that other complex policy programmes or initiatives will not encounter similar sorts of challenges, and there may be nothing here that is unique to collaborative endeavours. However, one of the major challenges for collaborations is whether the costs of evaluating these initiatives outweigh the results that they produce. We have, more than once, come across evaluations (or proposed evaluation plans) that would cost more than actually delivering the collaborative programme, which seems strange indeed.

Box 2.1: Some of the key challenges to consider when evaluating collaborations

- Collaboration takes many forms. If you are considering a comparative design (comparing collaborations), or seeking to be able to generalise from the data, are you sure you are comparing like with like?
- Collaborations bring together diverse groups. What do different stakeholders consider to be measures of the success of the collaboration, or what does success look like according to these different perspectives? How are these accounted for in the evaluation?
- How do the aims of the collaboration differ from previous arrangements and other improvement programmes?
- Where do the agendas of partners overlap and form joint work, and what falls outside this collaborative endeavour? In other words, what falls within the evaluation scope, and what is off limits?
- Which outcome measures are most appropriate to the aims and objectives of the collaboration?
- What aspects of the contexts have helped/hindered the formation and functioning of the collaboration?
- What are the chains of causality/theories underpinning the impact that the collaboration is intended to have? How can this map onto inputs, processes and outputs, and the various forms of outcomes?
- How can we capture and measure any unintended consequences of the collaboration?
- Over what timescale would you expect to see outcomes occur? Are these realistic/pragmatic?

- How can you be certain that any changes in outcomes are due to the collaboration and not other influences/policies in the local area? What controls can/cannot be built into the evaluation?
- Is your local population broadly similar to that at the start of the project? Are you measuring effects on individuals who have received services from the collaborative endeavour?
- How can you prove you have prevented something?
- What would have happened if you had not established the collaboration and had continued to deliver services in their previous form?

We have already established that collaboration can take a plethora of forms, and that we need to be careful when we draw lessons concerning the impact of collaboration or learning across initiatives. To this we can add that, by their nature, collaborations comprise a number of groups that may have different perspectives of what they should achieve, and consequently of how the partnership should be evaluated (Thomas and Palfrey, 1996). The key message here is that there is the potential for very different perspectives, not just between different collaborative initiatives, or from external scrutineers, but also from within the collaborative endeavour itself. For a further illustration of this, see Dickinson et al's (2013) study of joint commissioning where stakeholders within and across different collaborative arrangements thought about the potential impact of these arrangements in very different ways.

It would not be too far fetched to expect that partners should have at least one common goal. If you should find yourself in a situation where there is a collaborative arrangement between one or more partners who do not share at least one common goal, then you might want to rethink why it is that you have decided to work together. Beyond one or more shared goals, partners may have additional or different agendas that they have not necessarily shared with one another, or with the full set of parties to the collaboration. One of the great mistakes in collaborative working is to assume that partners have to do everything together – after all, if this is the case, why do you need two different entities? In order to effectively evaluate joint working it is important to think about where the overlaps of activity are and what doesn't fall within them. Although this sounds like a relatively straightforward step, as we will come back to at a number of points in this text, in practice this is less easy than it sounds. And yet, failing to recognise different concepts of success (see Huxham and Hibbert, 2008) leads to inappropriate conclusions about the effectiveness of collaborative working, and potentially to the inappropriate application of research results (Ouwens et al, 2005).

Given the multiplicity of definitions, forms and aims, there is no single set of outcome indicators that can be used to assess whether a collaborative endeavour has been successful. Drawing on evidence from the US, Schmitt (2001) suggests that what is often missing from evaluations of collaborative efforts is an explanation of why certain outcome indicators were selected to evaluate the impacts of collaboration. It might seem obvious that if we select an outcome around, say, efficiency or timeliness of services, but we aren't clear about why these have been selected and how this relates to the aims of the collaborative endeavour, we might not get the results we were seeking. Further, we may not be able to provide a fuller perspective of what the impact of collaboration is. A crucial first stage, then, in evaluating collaboration, is to identify the impacts you are seeking to measure and to be clear about how these link to the aims of the partnership. Having a frank discussion about what the collaboration is trying to achieve, how it will go about that, and how partners will know if these goals have been achieved, are important initial stages of collaborative endeavours.

Another key difference between collaborations is the context in which they operate. So that we can learn lessons about the functioning of a collaboration, we need to understand important facets of the setting in which it operates. It is important to recognise that what works in one situation may not in another (Pollitt, 1995) – developing general principles about successful collaboration is more difficult than it might seem. McNulty and Ferlie (2002) talk about the importance of 'receptive contexts' in terms of organisational change, and the evidence suggests that there can be much about context that influences successful and unsuccessful collaboration, such as the history of relationships (see Glasby and Dickinson, 2014, for a discussion of this; and O'Flynn et al, 2011, on relational capital in joined-up approaches) or the size of organisations and other potential competing local organisations (see Miller et al, 2011, for an exploration of this in relation to care trusts)

Bringing together the concepts of aspired outcomes and context leads us to a further challenge relating to the idea of attribution. This challenge is most often manifest where collaborations are aiming to address 'wicked' or complex social issues. In these cases we often find that different kinds of collaborative arrangements are seeking to address similar sorts of challenges (for example, reduce health inequalities, improve life chances for young children), and it can be difficult to identify which initiative has had what impact on these outcomes. When these various collaborative efforts are themselves not coordinated or connected, there can be considerable confusion in specific policy areas or even geographic places. It is not uncommon for collaborative arrangements to be tripping over each other in practice. Under the New Labour governments a whole range of government initiatives co-existed with broadly similar aims and often within the same kind of socioeconomically deprived areas, including Health Action Zones, Sure Start, New Deal for Communities, Education Action Zones, Children's Fund projects and so on. It was unclear how these various programmes coordinated between themselves, raising a governance and evaluation challenge. This is even more of a predicament when the causal links between action and impact are unclear, as illustrated in the case of LSPs, where evaluation reports argued that it was difficult to demonstrate clear outcomes because chains of causality were so complex (DfT, 2005, p 17). It may be the case that rather than clear links between intervention and outcome, the influence of collaborative work is subtle, indirect and cumulative, making it all the more difficult to capture in a concrete way.

Evaluations typically aim to capture all the impacts of an initiative, and this includes any potential unplanned or unintended consequences. There is the possibility that collaborative working arrangements might have an impact on the wider system (either positive or negative) that are unplanned and worth capturing. This process can be more challenging within very complex service delivery environments where it can be more difficult to establish all the impacts that working arrangements have on the broader environment. A further problem for evaluators of collaborative initiatives is to identify what would have happened if they had not worked collaboratively and had continued with more traditional arrangements. This is known as the challenge of the 'counter-factual', and is often dealt with through the creation of control groups (explained in more detail below).

In Chapter 1 we explained that we would make use of the Sure Start case study to demonstrate many of the issues that we talk about in this and other chapters, and we return to it here. Over the course of the evaluation of this programme a number of reports were produced. In one such report (Wiggins et al, 2005), it was found that there was little in terms of impact of the programme; in fact, some children were found to be worse off in the areas targeted by the scheme. It was suggested that while children of middle-class families did better, those of families in lower socioeconomic groups did worse. However, these observations didn't necessarily mean that the scheme wasn't working. Many of the targets that Sure Start is set up to achieve are long-term, and it could be argued that we would not expect to see the real impacts until the children in these areas reach the latter half of their teenage years.

When examining the impacts of long-term and wide-ranging programmes such as this, timescales often prove to be a tricky issue for evaluators. There is a substantial difference between expecting to see changes take place within short (more politically acceptable) timescales of, say, three years in comparison with the 15 years plus that it might actually take to demonstrate change in practice. In recent times the coalition government argued that the Troubled Families programme had not only 'turned around' 105,000 families, but had also saved taxpayers some £1.2 billion, despite the fact that the actual commissioned evaluations had not been completed. Critics were quick to pounce on the announcement, arguing: 'We have, as of now, absolutely no idea whether the TFP [Troubled Families programme] has saved taxpayers anything at all; and if it has, how much. The £1.2 billion is pure, unadulterated fiction' (Portes, 2015). An interesting international comparison can be found in Australia in its joined-up approach to addressing the systemic disadvantage of Indigenous peoples, and the challenge of long-term intergenerational social-economic outcomes and short-term reporting regimes (see Head and O'Flynn, 2015, for an in-depth discussion).

Box 2.2 sets out how *The Guardian* newspaper reported the early Sure Start findings. What is intriguing about this piece is that it is not only critical of either the programme or the evaluation. This might have a significant amount to do with the political views of this paper (and indeed the reporter), and to some extent the moment in time (it is unlikely that the current fiscal context would be quite so forgiving). What it does highlight nicely is the length of time it takes to fully realise the impacts of programmes like this, and the fact that this is often not compatible with the swift pace of political time frames.

There is another reason why we might have seen a lack of impact in socioeconomically deprived areas. Often research finds that where programmes help individuals and families overcome some significant challenges, an early activity can be to seek to move out of that area. This family may be replaced by another with a fresh range of challenging issues to contend with. In other words, although the population remains constant and might reflect similar trends at a macro scale, this is actually hiding some quite significant changes at the micro level. With large-scale evaluations such as this it is important to take this factor into account, and to make sure that when doing comparative analysis the same individuals are being compared with each other over time. This example further illustrates the difficulties in attempting to generalise the impacts of quite different local programmes, which all exist within particular contexts and have different ranges of alternative services available to children and families.

Box 2.2: Media report on the early impacts of Sure Start

[P]erversely, children of teenage mothers seemed to do worse in Sure Start areas. But the programme has been dealt a blow; experts, including those who did the study, agree the problem lies in the hard-to-measure design of Sure Start and in government pressure for early results. How can you prove a miracle effect on the hardest-to-change children when the first Sure Starts had been open only 18 months? Researchers compared 19,000 under-fives, half in Sure Start areas, the rest from similarly deprived districts, but found no discernible developmental, language or behavioural differences. Crucially, they were not asked to compare children actually in Sure Start programmes, only those living in the area, many of whom had no contact with it....

The scheme was set unrealistically tough targets – such as reducing the number of low-birthweight babies in the area. But the key test was whether children progressed faster. Experts advising on the evaluation warned that effective results would come only when the same children were followed for years. But politics doesn't work to academic timetables....The ambiguous results were not the fault of the eminent researchers, whose problems were legion. Poor areas have a high turnover of families; Enfield Sure Start ... had an 80% turnover of under-fives, so any evaluation missed many children with a lot of Sure Start help who moved away, while catching newcomers who might have had none.

No complex social scheme makes for a crisp laboratory experiment, but ministers yearned for hard proof that would cement Sure Start into the welfare state. The control areas also had schemes and action zones; indeed, places without Sure Start often had better help for some groups, such as teenage mothers. Sure Start areas were assumed to be reaching this group, though many were not. Researchers didn't know how many children in either group had what help, if any.

Every Sure Start is different, run variously by health, education and voluntary groups or local authorities: the original ethos was to let a thousand flowers bloom. They are so popular partly because mothers have a big say in how local schemes are run. But without a fixed template, the same everywhere, researchers couldn't know what they were measuring.

Sure Start was inspired by Head Start, a US programme for deprived under-fives. Results of one part showed how every $1 spent on under-fives saved $7 by the time the children were 30; they committed fewer crimes, had fewer mental problems, drew less social security and had better jobs and qualifications. But in the early years Head Start also produced little measurable effect. It wasn't until their teens that Head Start children pulled away, apparently better protected from adolescent problems.

Here is one piece of early encouragement. The one positive finding in this Sure Start study may prove vital in the long run – Sure Start mothers give "warmer parenting" than the control group, with less hostility, less smacking, less negative criticism and more affection. That has not translated so far into improvement in children's progress, but academics expect it to augur well for emotional and social development.

Source: Polly Toynbee, *The Guardian* (Tuesday 13 September 2005)

What should collaborative working achieve in theory?

So far this chapter has argued that the evidence suggests that there is little agreement on the impact of collaboration on outcomes. One possible explanation for this is that, even if we set aside the complex social interventions being undertaken, collaboration itself is difficult to evaluate, and there has been a tendency to privilege process over outcome evaluation in this field. This section explores what collaborative working should achieve according to the theory. After all, one of the first stages in evaluating collaborative working is to determine what impact we think it should produce, so it is worth going to the more theoretical literature to establish what some of the potential effects might be.

As outlined in the introductory text in this series (Glasby and Dickinson, 2014), it has long been suggested that services are typically organised in one of three ways: hierarchies, markets and networks. *Hierarchies* tend to be a single organisation (perhaps a large bureaucracy), with top-down rules, procedures and statutes that govern how the organisation works. In contrast, *markets* involve organisations exchanging goods and services based on competition and price. *Networks* are often seen as lying in between these two approaches, with multiple organisations coming together more informally, often based on interpersonal relationships or a shared outlook (Thompson, 1991; 6 et al, 2006). A *transaction cost economics* perspective of these forms (for example, Williamson, 1975) suggests that when organisations are forced to collaborate, selection of one form over another is based on the nature of the product or service being produced, the ability to predict the actions of a partner and the efficiency implications of these factors.

The following analysis of this perspective builds on that set out in Glasby and Dickinson (2014), expanding on this brief account in more detail so that we might have a clear sense of the different reasons why organisations collaborate and what these processes should result in.

Markets are effective when the value of a good is certain (that is, it is fixed and not open to contest) and a contract can be used to ensure delivery of that good (with legal backing). Yet where there is uncertainty over value, some form of hierarchy may be a more efficient way of making transactions between its members than a market. In a hierarchy, each party works towards the aims of the organisation, which places a value on each contribution and compensates it fairly. As the organisation is trusted in this relationship, the transaction costs are lower, overcoming some of the difficulties markets have with collaboration.

However, due to the formalisation and routine of hierarchies, these lower transaction costs tend to come at the price of flexibility.

Networks tend to be characterised by actors recognising complementary interests and developing interdependent relationships based on trust, loyalty and reciprocity to enable and maintain collaborative activity (for a discussion on multiparty networks in service delivery, see Alford and O'Flynn, 2012). In an ideal situation, network actors are working towards the same aims and objectives and therefore generate trust between each other. This trust reduces transaction costs without creating the same formal structures associated with hierarchies (although actors will be bound by informal rules). In these trust-based networks partners can work together more effectively as they perceive less uncertainty between stakeholders and can better predict the actions of their partners (Rowlinson, 1997; Putnam, 2003). Underpinning this analysis is the notion that efficiency ultimately determines what form of collaboration organisations enter into.

As useful as the analysis of markets, hierarchies and networks is, it tells us more about the form that collaboration takes, rather than the reason for this collaboration. In other words, this analysis presupposes that collaboration is necessary, and then suggests the most efficient way of carrying out these interactions given particular features of the context. Moreover, as 6 et al (2006) note, in reality organisations tend not to exist in these essentialist forms, but to be a settlement between one or more of these ways of organising. For example, networks operating in practice often have characteristics of markets and hierarchies, are centralised, and may not be so trust-based (Alford and O'Flynn, 2012). Drawing on Challis et al's (1988) work on optimist and pessimist perspectives of collaboration, Sullivan and Skelcher (2002, p 36) developed a framework that incorporates a range of approaches to understanding collaboration, based on 'optimistic', 'pessimistic' and 'realistic' perspectives of collaboration (outlined in Table 2.1), and these are explained in further detail below.

Table 2.1: Optimist, pessimist and realist theories of collaboration

	Optimist	Pessimist	Realist
Why collaboration happens?	Achieving shared vision: *Collaborative empowerment theory Regime theory* Resource maximisation: *Exchange theory*	Maintaining/ enhancing position: *Resource dependency theory*	Responding to new environments: *Evolutionary theory*
What form of collaboration is developed and why?	Multiple relationships: *Collaborative empowerment theory*	Interorganisational network: *Resource dependency theory*	Formalised networks: *Evolutionary theory* Policy networks as governance instruments: *Policy networks theories*

Optimist perspectives

Optimist perspectives of collaboration tend to be characterised as those that presuppose consensus and shared vision between partners. They suggest that partners collaborate to produce positive results for the entire system, and predominantly for altruistic purposes. One such example is *exchange theory*. Implicit in this concept of collaboration is that by working together organisations may achieve more than they may do separately, that is, 'synergy' or 'collaborative advantage'. Exchange theory, as suggested by Levine and White (1962), states that organisations collaborate as they are dependent on each other for *resources*. Partners *voluntarily* choose to interact as they are dependent on the resources of other organisations in order to achieve their overall goals or objectives.

Regime theory (see, for example, Stoker, 1995) is another example, arguing that organisations from the public, private and third sectors come together to accomplish long-term gains for the good of the wider system, although this is not necessarily an entirely altruistic process. For example, private businesses may get involved in city-wide regeneration initiatives as, in the long run, the increased attractiveness of the city where this company is based may pay off financially or provide these businesses with a stronger voice. *Collaborative betterment* and *collaborative empowerment* (see, for example, Himmelman, 1996, 2001) theories, meanwhile, are interested in collaboration between the state and citizens, and about more actively involving citizens in decision-making processes.

Pessimist perspectives

Pessimist perspectives of collaboration predict that organisations or agencies will only enter into such arrangements if they enhance their own gain or power above anything else. In other words, the process of collaboration will only occur if it is in the mutual interest of each party to try to control or influence the other's activities. Other writers have discussed how parties 'fail' into collaboration as a last resort, when nothing else seems to work (see O'Flynn, 2009). One example of this approach is *resource dependency theory* (RDT). Although RDT is credited to the work of Pfeffer and Salancik (1978), Emerson (1962) noted that social relationships often involve ties of mutual dependence, meaning actors are dependent on the resources controlled by another to achieve their desired goals. Power lies in the dependency of actors on each other. RDT proposes that actors lacking in essential resources will seek to establish relationships with (that is, be dependent on) others in order to obtain needed resources. Organisations attempt to alter their dependence relationships by minimising their own dependence or by increasing the dependence of other organisations on them.

Realist perspectives

Sullivan and Skelcher (2002) added the 'realist' perspective category to the optimist and pessimist viewpoints. In the context of a text dealing with the issue of evaluation it is important to note that this 'realist' perspective should not be confused with a realist philosophy of research, which we explore in more detail throughout the text. Realist philosophy holds a realist ontology (that is, an understanding about the nature of the world), which proposes that things exist independently of our consciousness of them, as opposed to perspectives that suggest the socially constructed nature of the world (see Dickinson and Carey, 2016). The realist perspectives that Sullivan and Skelcher refer to is not this philosophy, but a more nuanced view of the reasons why collaboration might exist than the optimist and pessimist perspectives outlined above, suggesting that in response to the wider environment, altruism and individual gain may coexist. The crux of this perspective is how organisations change in response to the wider environment, and how they might achieve either (or both) gains through collaboration. One theory that sets out this position, and which is often implicitly alluded to in much recent health and social care policy, is *evolutionary theory* (see below). Alter and Hage (1993) suggest that collaboration is becoming more likely due to a variety of reasons, including changing political and economic objectives; changing technological capacity; and an increasing demand for quality and diversity in services. In other words, evolutionary theory suggests that agencies are forced to collaborate due to changes in the external environment. These changes have the potential both to increase the power of resources over other agencies and to produce beneficial effects for those who use these services.

A further theory that might broadly come under the banner of 'realist' perspectives is that of *new institutional theory*. A number of the theories outlined above suggest that collaboration is introduced as a response to changes in the external environment. Institutional theory examines why organisations might see collaboration as a valid solution, but do so not from the perspective of material goods (for example, money), but due to cultural factors. DiMaggio and Powell (1991) suggest that the emergent belief system about organisations supersedes any possible beliefs about the most effective ways of arranging particular organisational aspects. For neo-institutional theorists, the current enthusiasm for collaboration might partly be explained by the phenomenon of institutional isomorphism. Put simply, this means that organisations enter into collaborative working arrangements because collaboration is inscribed with value in their normative environment.

In other words, organisations take on particular characteristics or initiatives, not because they have necessarily demonstrated that they are the most effective, but because the institutional environment values these behaviours. This point is of particular interest in relation to collaboration, given the enthusiasm with which this agenda has been welcomed nationally and internationally. O'Flynn (2014) describes how collaboration has emerged as the *modus operandi* of 21st-century public services, the 'one best way' to organise. Broad reading on the topic shows that collaboration is often positioned as the answer to any number of different questions despite a lack of clear evidence to suggest that this is an effective solution. (This theme is explored in further detail in Chapter 3, in relation to the performance of collaboration.) Oliver (1990) provides a summary of what he argues are the six main reasons why collaborations are established (see Box 2.3; see also O'Flynn, 2014, for the various 'stories' or imperatives for joined-up approaches). As we can see from this there are several potential drivers of collaboration, and many of these fall more firmly into the pessimistic or realistic than optimistic categories. Much of the rhetoric of collaboration in health and social care is about the importance of designing and providing services around citizens (echoing themes in exchange theory and evolutionary theory), promising to tackle complex problems and produce 'collaborative advantage' (Kanter, 1994). Policy consistently asserts that partners can achieve more together than they can do apart, although they often lack clarity in terms of what this advantage looks like.

The theme of efficiency that is strongly present in many of the theories outlined above has often been less explicitly discussed with respect to collaborative working. Although there are a number of experiments with joint funding mechanisms (Mason et al, 2015), and efficiency has become an ever-more important theme since the global financial crisis and recent governments' reductions in public service funding, it is unusual to see efficiency being cited as a sole driver of collaborative working in health and social care. What is interesting here is that although we know from the theoretical material that the need to share and/or control resources is an important driver, it is one that is rarely cited on its own as being an important reason for collaborative working.

Box 2.3: Six reasons why collaborations are established

- *Necessity:* that is, partnerships are mandated by law or regulation.
- *Asymmetry:* one party wishes to exercise control over another.
- *Reciprocity:* partners seek mutual benefit through cooperation.
- *Efficiency:* partners may gain more efficiency through cooperation.
- *Stability:* organisations can encounter less uncertainty through interaction.
- *Legitimacy:* organisations may obtain or enhance their public image through cooperation.

Source: Oliver (1990)

What can we understand from this situation? One suggestion could be that public service collaboration is driven by a range of factors. After all, many of the theories and models around collaboration have been developed in relation to the private sector, and these might not be so clearly applicable to public service settings. Another suggestion might be that policy and health and social care organisations are not always explicit about the drivers of collaborative working. If health and social care organisations justify activity in terms of efficiency dividends alone, they run the risk of paying attention to inputs and outputs and not the level of care or quality of services. In these cases, policy and professionals may draw more attention to patient outcomes and service quality than efficiency – even if the latter is a major aim (and, after all, making services more efficient should release more money to reinvest in services). The final reason we offer is that there is often an implicit assumption that collaboration will produce better services and better outcomes, without ever being entirely clear about how, or what, this will look like in practice. Collaboration is often assumed to be a 'good thing' or, as McLaughlin (2004, p 103) writes, 'to argue for the importance of partnerships is like arguing for "mother love and apple pie". The notion of partnership working has an inherently positive moral feel about it and it has become almost heretical to question its integrity.' Indeed, some have gone as far as to argue that there is a 'cult of collaboration' (O'Flynn, 2009).

One of the challenges here is that without a sense of which drivers are present, it is difficult to be clear about whether this collaboration has achieved success or not. Of course, in reality, collaboration may be driven by several factors (see O'Flynn, 2014, for a discussion of imperatives). For example, under the Health Act 1999 health and social care organisations have a legal duty to cooperate with one another (*necessity*), but specific partnerships might be set up to reduce duplication between agencies (*efficiency*), while also producing more seamless solutions for specific service user groups (*reciprocity*), allowing the local authority to exert more power over the activities of a local clinical commissioning group (CCG) (*asymmetry*), and also offering the CCG more legitimacy through the accountability structures of the local authority (*legitimacy*). To complicate matters further, different stakeholders within organisations might hold a variety of beliefs concerning what the collaboration is driven by, and these may or may not accord with the beliefs of others. What all of this tells us is that it is important that we are clear about what is driving the specific collaboration, and what success will look like for this specific arrangement. It is to this topic we now turn.

Importance of clarity over the drivers and outcomes of collaboration

So far we have made the argument that collaboration is often assumed to be a positive thing that health and social care communities should be involved in. By and large this is the image painted by the literature on collaboration. However, some have drawn attention to the negatives of working collaboratively. For Alex Scott-Samuel, collaborative working is described as setting aside 'mutual loathing' in order to get your hands on someone else's money (quoted in Powell and Dowling, 2006, p 308). Given the theoretical literature on collaboration where resource dependency is presented as an important driver, we can see why Scott-Samuel might suggest this. Scott-Samuel is not the only commentator to draw attention to the potential negative effects of collaborative working, and this theme is explored further in the introductory book in this series (see Glasby and Dickinson, 2014). Lundin (2007) argued that, in the wrong situations, joint working could be both unhelpful and costly, and Huxham (1996, p 3), an internationally recognised expert on collaboration, argues that 'most of what organizations strive to achieve is, and should be, done alone.' In later work with Siv Vangen, the key message was made very clearly: 'don't work collaboratively unless you have to' (Huxham and Vangen, 2004, p 200).

Even government agencies, usually very positive about working together, have drawn attention to the potential negative impacts of collaborative working. The Audit Commission, for example, warned that:

> Partnerships also bring risks. Working across organisational boundaries brings complexity and ambiguity that can generate confusion and weaken accountability. The principle of accountability for public money applies as much to partnerships as to corporate bodies. The public needs assurance that public money is spent wisely in partnerships and it should be confident that its quality of life will improve

as a result of this form of working. (Audit Commission, 2005, p 2)

The important point here is that we should not assume that collaborative working will bring only positive outcomes – it can be a complex process, and we need to be mindful of ensuring the same sorts of standards of accountability as we would with other forms of working relationships. So far in this chapter we have argued that there are many drivers for collaboration, local arrangements are not as clear as they might be about the outcomes that they are trying to deliver through collaborative working, and collaborative endeavours can also result in zero or even negative impact. Added to these observations is the idea covered in Chapter 1, that there is a range of different reasons why we might evaluate our activities. If collaboration and evaluation can be driven by many different factors and achieve different kinds of outcomes, it is important that we are clear about the particular drivers of any collaborative working arrangement and the outcomes that we aspire to. If this is lacking, local collaborative arrangements may find that it is difficult to assess the degree to which they have been successful. Local collaborations may also find that different stakeholder groups hold varied perspectives about what initiatives should achieve, and if this is not reflected in terms of activity, they will become disenchanted with the collaboration over time. Box 2.4 provides an overview of a case study where there was lack of clarity over the drivers and intended outcomes of collaborative working.

From the research presented in Box 2.4, Dickinson and Glasby add two additional categories to the drivers of collaborative working set out by Sullivan and Skelcher (2002) earlier. To optimist, pessimist and realist they add pragmatist and mimetist. To the pragmatist, collaborative working sounds like a positive concept, which is difficult for critics to argue against. The concept of collaboration is used in this context as it is assumed that other stakeholders may object if the real organisational drivers were stated. In these circumstances we find that political and organisational drivers are justified in terms of positive outcomes for staff and/or service users. According to a mimetist perspective, collaboration is an automatic policy response to a problem – others are doing this and it generally seems to be expected. Although we may not be sure about the specific outcomes expected, working together in some way is understood to be a good thing; not to be collaborating would be seen as being out of step with current practice. There is a desire to improve services, but it is an imprecise and slightly naive approach, without being clear about the desired outcomes.

Box 2.4: Forensic Mental Health Partnership and the importance of clarity over drivers and outcomes

Dickinson and Glasby (2010) set out an account of a partnership between a specialist forensic mental health trust, Springfield Mental Health Trust, and a more generalist mental health trust, Shelbyville Mental Health Trust in England. Springfield is nationally renowned, financially robust, and seen as a leading provider of care, while Shelbyville is smaller, based out of town, provides more community-based services, and has previously received negative reports from healthcare inspectors about some aspects of the quality of care it provides. These two trusts formed the Forensic Mental Health Partnership (FMHP), which involved Shelbyville staff working in forensics transferring their employment to Springfield, the lead partner managing the overall forensic services provided at both sites. The arrangement was deliberately presented from the start to staff, service users and other stakeholders as a 'partnership', where there would be mutual learning and sharing in directions between the two organisations. Shelbyville would benefit from the expertise, reputation and resources of Springfield, that would, in turn, learn about community-based services.

However, the research that Dickinson and Glasby undertook a year after FMHP had been established suggested that it was perceived not as a 'partnership' but as a 'takeover'. Many of the front-line staff at Shelbyville were unhappy with this, feeling that it should be a partnership of equals. Yet in terms of how FMHP had been established, it did seem that Springfield was performing a takeover: they were the dominant group of staff on the board; all meetings took place at the Springfield site; and those at Shelbyville felt disowned by their own organisation now that their management had been delegated to Springfield. The procedures, approach and culture of FMHP were all perceived to be Springfield-dominated, with little of Shelbyville visible.

Further, FMHP staff found it difficult to be clear about the types of outcomes it was that they were aiming to achieve through the partnership. While they agreed it was about better services and being more innovative, on closer interrogation many of the aspirations were about the more efficient use of scarce resources (for example, single point of access, preventing duplication, simplifying procedures), or were altogether vastly aspirational and well beyond the stated remit of the partnership (for example, bring in more interpreters, 'sort out' another hospital in the local area not involved in the partnership, improve the health of children in the city as a whole, create better relationships with the local authority who again were not a partner). Although the brochures and publicity material talked very much about FMHP being driven by service user outcomes, the overriding impression from staff was that FMHP was designed to benefit partner organisations. This was further confirmed when in interviews senior managers suggested that part of the initial motivation had come from both organisations attempting to respond to local and national political issues.

As Dickinson and Glasby outline:

> At the time the Partnership was first discussed, Shelbyville had recently experienced a high profile mental health homicide and a very critical serious case review was expected shortly. Also at this time, the region was reviewing the current configuration of mental health services, and Shelbyville was one of the organizations rumoured to be at risk of closure or merger. Meanwhile, Springfield was fighting hard to throw off a reputation of being aloof and autocratic, arguing that it should be at the centre of a regional mental health system. Against this background, FMHP was a timely development, as it gave important messages to national policy makers that Shelbyville was dedicated to improving its services and that Springfield

> was working hard to be a more collaborative member of its local and regional health community. (2010, p 818)

Staff at Shelbyville had essentially bought into FMHP as they fundamentally believed that a 'true' partnership would mean that there would be sharing across the organisations, and therefore that staff and service users alike would benefit. Further, staff believed that this would not simply offer a way of sharing across organisations, but would also fulfil a range of fantastical outcomes that went well beyond the remit of the managerial relationship between the hospitals. Staff never questioned the notion that a partnership might not mean mutual sharing and could involve a takeover. Publically, the organisational drivers identified above were not articulated, but they were certainly dominant in the rationale for the establishment of the partnership. Calling the arrangement a 'partnership' helped win staff over and establish the FMHP, which involved significant change to processes of accountability, finance and human resources, changes that could not be easily reversed when staff realised they were unhappy with the outcome.

As this example illustrates, publically articulating a case around one set of drivers and aspired outcomes when they are actually driven by other factors can, at the very least, result in a disengagement of professionals from the overall aims of the organisation. In Jelphs et al (2016) there is more detail about the importance of a clear set of aspirations to the process of teamwork, and this lesson is important to consider in terms of collaborative working more broadly. If collaboration endeavours are justified on one basis (for example, improving services) but really about another (for example, cutting costs), we should not be surprised if individuals disengage from this agenda. Such an approach also makes evaluation difficult – what should be evaluated – the publicly stated purpose (for example, improved services) or the actual purpose (for example, reduced costs)? If we focus on the formally articulated drivers and aspirations, it should be no surprise that an evaluation will likely show unimpressive results; after all, the collaboration isn't really intended to have an impact on these factors. Research into the outcomes of the joint commissioning process in England by Dickinson et al (2013) found that those sites that were able to articulate a clear sense of the drivers for collaborative working and their intended aspirations were more able to mobilise their workforce towards these goals and to demonstrate their impact to a variety of different audiences. A clear mission can, in practice, motivate actors (Alford and O'Flynn, 2012). This process, in turn, provided local organisations with a greater mandate for operational and evaluative activity going forward.

Torbay Care Trust provides another example relating to a site that clearly kept the aspirations of the outcomes in mind when structuring day-to-day activities. In this example, the trust used a fictional person representing the average service user – Mrs Smith – as a central focus in decision-making processes. This person-centred approach built incrementally over time, as professionals considered how delivery could benefit this service user. Where changes did not promise to improve things for Mrs Smith, they were reconsidered (Thistlethwaite, 2011). A key lesson to take from this chapter is the need to be clear within a certain degree about what a collaborative endeavour has been set up to achieve, why this is seen as the best course of action, and the sorts of outcomes it is aiming to achieve. Moreover, evaluations need to reflect the everyday difficulties that those working within partnerships encounter, or else they run the risk of being disregarded by the very people who stand to learn the most from these findings.

Reflective exercises

1. Think about a collaboration you have experience of or have read about. What are the key drivers for collaborating in that case? What would success look like in that example?
2. Compare two policy documents that advocate for collaborative working. What drivers do they talk about? Are these similar or different sorts of drivers?
3. Thinking about the same example you used in the previous chapter, how would you go about evaluating this collaboration? What are the main difficulties you might encounter in this process?
4. Think about a collaboration that involves a wide range of different stakeholders (for example, health, social care, voluntary and community sector groups, education, leisure services and so on). Do you think that all partner organisations hold the same vision of what 'success' would look like? How might opinions differ?

Further reading and resources

- For a good introduction to issues around public policy collaboration and theoretical drivers of partnership, see Sullivan and Skelcher's (2002) *Working across boundaries* and O'Flynn, et al (2014) 'You win some, you lose some: Experiments with joined-up government'.
- In addition to Sure Start, there are a range of national evaluations of partnership initiatives that have useful lessons about the evaluation process, including:
  - the Children's Fund (Edwards et al, 2006)
  - children's trusts (University of East Anglia, 2007)
  - Health Act flexibilities (Glendinning et al, 2002)
  - Health Action Zones (Barnes et al, 2005)
  - intermediate care (Barton et al, 2005)
  - local area agreements (ODPM, 2005a, 2007)
  - LSPs (ODPM, 2005b)
  - *National evaluation of the Department of Health's Integrated Care Pilots* (RAND Europe and Ernst & Young, 2012)

- – *Joint commissioning in health and social care* (Dickinson et al, 2013)
- – *National evaluation of the Troubled Families programme* (DCLG, 2014).
- For an interesting international comparison, see the Closing the Gap strategy in Australia, which centres on a national partnership agreement (between national, state and territory governments) to address the disadvantage of Indigenous peoples in Australia. A good overview is provided in Head and O'Flynn (2015), and more detailed information is set out here: www.coag.gov.au/closing_the_gap_in_indigenous_disadvantage

3

Hot topics and emerging issues

This chapter explores a series of tensions around the evaluation of health and social care collaboration in more detail, focusing on some specific areas of debate within the literature, including:

- How can collaboration be effectively evaluated?
- What kinds of evidence about integration might we present to different groups?
- Performing governance: what is the additional work of collaboration?

How can collaboration be effectively evaluated?

In Chapter 2 we argued that evaluating collaboration can be a difficult process. Gomez-Bonnet and Thomas (2015, p 28) explain that 'methods to evaluate partnerships have ... proliferated, but tend to focus only on particular aspects of partnerships. None alone provide a comprehensive picture of how a partnership is working.' In this section we explore some of the different approaches that have been used to evaluate collaborative working, and the appropriateness of these to particular purposes and settings. This section provides background in terms of methodology and philosophy of evaluation to consider the frameworks and tools that will be set out in the following chapter. We start by setting out the methodology adopted in the Sure Start programme that we have already spoken about in the previous two chapters (see Box 3.1). As this illustrates, the Sure Start evaluation was composed of different components, each devised to analyse different issues. For each of these components it was decided what was under investigation and which approach would be most suited to uncovering these factors. As this demonstrates, approaches were formative and summative, quantitative and qualitative, and the various components of the national study were used to reinforce and inform other strands. In this way the evaluation was able to incorporate local and national, process and outcome (intermediate and long-term) evaluations, to compare these with other areas and to track trends over time. It is important to note, however, that this is an expensive (£20 million) and long-term evaluation, which may not be suitable for all contexts. We explore the detail of many of these approaches in the remainder of this section.

Box 3.1: National Evaluation of Sure Start methodological approach

There were five components to the National Evaluation of Sure Start:

- *Implementation evaluation:* sought to illuminate the contents of the Sure Start 'black box'. Formative in nature, this aimed to produce a comprehensive picture of the processes and components of the first 260 programmes. Used quantitative (national questionnaire survey) and qualitative methods (in-depth case studies of 26 programmes).
- *Impact evaluation:* examined the effects of Sure Start on children, families and communities to identify the conditions under which Sure Start was most effective. Cross-sectional, longitudinal study comparing Sure Start programmes with randomly selected control communities. Large-scale quantitative study involving range of factors such as demographic, community, economic, health, development and service indicators.
- *Local community context analysis:* analysing the nature and patterns of Sure Start neighbourhoods. Used a range of data, from existing administrative databases, observations made by evaluators conducting interviews and questionnaires, to give an in-depth overview of the important factors and local-specific processes going on within these communities.
- *Cost-benefit analysis:* measured the relationship between costs of Sure Start and other services for children and families in Sure Start areas and the outcomes achieved (both intermediate and long-term). Cost-

benefit analysis was conducted for different groups of beneficiaries and different types of benefits.

- *Support for local evaluations:* investigated how local evaluators planned to evaluate local programmes and provided web- and workshop-based support and information exchange to these individuals.

Source: National Evaluation of Sure Start (2002)

The tendency of evaluations of collaborative working in health and social care to date has been to focus on the processes of collaborative working rather than on outcomes, partly because evaluating outcomes is more difficult than examining processes. As a consequence we have far more evidence about how partners can work together and the kinds of processes and practices that need to be in place than we do about the impact that these activities have in terms of outcomes for service users. It does not follow that what we need to do is simply focus on issues of outcomes in future evaluations to fill this evidence gap. There are many factors at play within collaborative working that may have a potential impact on the outcomes that these working arrangements produce. For example, interactions between individuals are an important dimension of how collaborations function (Gajda, 2004). Without knowing what is happening within a collaborative working arrangement, we can't say whether it is operating in a way that we would expect it to in order to produce particular impacts.

If we just examine the inputs and outputs/outcomes of a collaborative endeavour and try to draw lessons from this, we may get an incomplete picture of the situation. In the evaluation literature this is known as a 'black box' approach, as we lack information about what is happening in terms of the operation of the collaboration. Evaluations that incorporate an overview of internal processes, that seek to open up the black box, are often referred to as 'clear' or 'white box' evaluations (see Figure 3.1). The difference in these approaches is their treatment of causality. In black box evaluations causality is inferred from observing conjunctions of inputs, outputs and outcomes (that is, if we put in x, we observe that we get y out, which has z effect,

Figure 3.1: Black box and 'clear box' evaluations

Black box evaluation: little information on processes taking place within partnership, need to infer causality

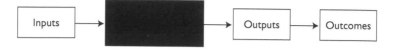

Clear box evaluation: processes mapped out, can make statements about causality with more certainty

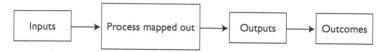

therefore we presume that x causes y and z). Clear box evaluations aim to observe these causal chains in more detail and make more definitive statements about the nature of these relationships – we know, with a reasonable degree of certainty, that x is strongly linked with y and z, rather than just being generally associated with these factors. Where we do not know for certain that particular mechanisms lead to certain effects, evaluators often seek to map out inputs, processes, outputs and outcomes in order that they may be able to say with certainty which sorts of activities delivered particular forms of impacts.

As an example of a clear box evaluation taken from the collaboration literature, Asthana et al (2003) formed a framework to inform their evaluation of Health Action Zones (set out in Figure 3.2). As we can see from this figure, the research team aimed to map out all of the assumptions about important factors in terms of the inputs, processes, outcomes and impacts, but also those in the context or principles of working arrangements that may have implications for the functioning of collaboration. In recent years we have seen the emergence of many more complex frameworks such as that set out by Asthana et al, representing a turn in interest towards theory-based approaches to evaluation. We briefly consider the difference between method-led and theory-led evaluation approaches, and their implications for analysing collaborative working.

Figure 3.2: A framework for examining partnership working

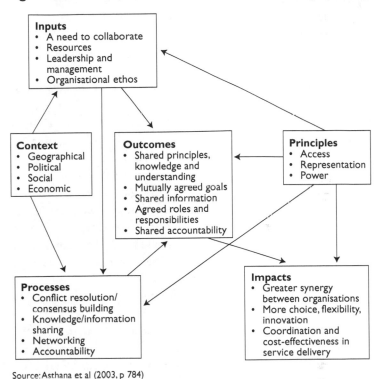

Source: Asthana et al (2003, p 784)

Method-led evaluation approaches

In Chapter 1 we noted that long-standing debates have argued over the relative merits of quantitative and qualitative approaches to evaluation. Broadly speaking, within the evaluation of collaborative working, quantitative methods have tended to be used to produce broadly generaliseable results over a fairly large population, but are unable to highlight individual differences over any large group (as the Sure Start example illustrated). Qualitative approaches are more able to accommodate such differences, but are much more resource-intensive, and as a result are likely to incorporate smaller sample sizes. All evaluations inevitably involve a series of trade-offs regarding what sort of coverage is gained, whose perspectives to involve and the main focus of the study. Not every evaluation will be able to cover every possibility, and even those that are large-scale and well funded (such as the Sure Start example) inevitably encounter some sort of negotiations. Typically the decision about whether to adopt a qualitative or quantitative approach in practice is a pragmatic one, dependent on the size, scale and purpose of the evaluation. Where we find complex evaluation approaches (again, like the Sure Start example) we typically see the use of mixed methods – quantitative and qualitative approaches combined to gain depth and breadth of perspective.

The debate over the relative merit of quantitative or qualitative approaches is broadly based around methodological issues. The method-led evaluation literature argues that where we see problems it is due to methodological shortcomings. According to this perspective, if we can just refine our research methods we should be able to address these issues (Chen, 1990). Table 3.1 sets out a broad overview of the main method-led approaches that have been used to evaluate collaboration in health and social care with a description of the strengths and weaknesses of these approaches.

One of the limitations of these approaches is that collaborative projects are increasingly oriented around 'wicked' issues that are multifaceted, complex and involving many actors. In these cases if we treat the collaborative programme as an on-off switch, we have to distinguish its effects from all the other factors that could lead to an on-off result (Patton, 1997; Weiss, 1999). In response to the challenges that arise over demonstrating the attribution of particular activities and their impacts, over the past 20 years theory-led approaches to evaluation have become increasingly popular.

Table 3.1: Method-led evaluation approaches

| Non-randomised comparative design | Seeks to control a number of variants in order to isolate relationships between the variables that are the subject of the study. Only by exerting such experimental control can the observer be confident that any relationships observed are meaningful and not due to extraneous forces. Compares outcomes for two sites selected to be as similar as possible in characteristics or two time periods for same site | Seeks to eradicate as much bias as possible through experimental approaches Can cover large service user groups Ability to generalise results | Failure to unlock the 'black box' and assess the processes within the partnership leading to attribution issues Difficulties associated with identifying homogeneous groups Problems in identifying unintended consequences | Comparison of clinical outcomes of patients served by integrated health and social care teams and more 'traditional' GP primary health arrangements (Levin et al, 2002; Brown et al, 2003; Davey et al, 2005) |

(continued)

Table 3.1: Method-led evaluation approaches (continued)

Approach	Brief description	Strengths	Limitations in practice	Example studies
Qualitative methods	Tend to take more grounded approaches to research, for example through interviews and case studies of individuals and families. Such approaches tend to reject the 'naive realism' often associated with quantitative methods. That is, a belief that there is a single, unequivocal social reality or truth which is entirely independent of the researcher and of the research process; instead there are multiple perspectives of the world that are created and constructed in the research process (Lincoln and Guba, 1985)	Accommodates multiple user perspectives In-depth account of process and context issues	Quite labour intensive, studies tend to be unable to incorporate large numbers of users with same resources as quantitative approaches Difficulties in generalising results to other groups Attribution difficulties; individuals unable to identify actions and policies and their direct effects	Evaluation of multiagency organisations working for disabled children with complex healthcare needs to assess their impact on professionals, families and the users (Townsley et al, 2004; Abbott et al, 2005)

(continued)

Table 3.1: Method-led evaluation approaches (continued)

Approach	Brief description	Strengths	Limitations in practice	Example studies
Multimethod approach	Combines both quantitative and qualitative approaches to gain the advantages of both types of approaches. However, such an approach often involves the researcher hopping from one epistemological base (or theory of knowledge) to another (Chen, 1990; Pawson and Tilley, 1997)	'A simultaneous multilevel multi-method (quantitative and qualitative) approach to research on partnerships is optimal, thus drawing on differing frameworks and seeking to embrace the perspective of all stakeholders and the complexity of the phenomena under study' (El Ansari and Weiss, 2006, p 178)	Such an approach does not necessarily overcome issues of attribution. Epistemological inconsistencies. Difficulties of consolidating data from different frameworks. Which stakeholder perspectives should be accepted?	Evaluation of the first combined mental health and social care provider in the UK, Somerset Partnership NHS and Social Care Trust (Peck et al, 2002)

Source: Dickinson (2006, p 377)

Theory-led evaluation approaches

The critique that theory-led evaluation approaches make of their method-led counterparts is that they tend to maximise one type of validity at the expense of others (Davies, 2000). Rather than inferring causation from the input and outputs of a project, theory-led evaluation aims to map out the entire process (Pawson and Tilley, 1997) and produce clear box evaluations. This then allows the researcher to say with confidence which parts of the collaboration worked and why, whether they would be applicable to different situations, and if there are any positive or negative effects that would otherwise not be anticipated (Birckmayer and Weiss, 2000). Such an approach is also helpful in respect to one of the challenges that we spent some time discussing in Chapter 2 – the importance of clarity in terms of the drivers and outcomes of collaborative working. Theory-based approaches demand that individuals and groups set out the full range of assumptions and aims that underpin a programme or activity in order to understand the processes at play within any context.

In practice, theory-led approaches adopt the kinds of methods we saw outlined above. What is different are not the tools of data collection, but the philosophy underpinning the approach to evaluation, with theory-led approaches being primarily interested in mid-range programme theory. In other words, theory-led approaches start from the perspective that within complex interventions it is not always clear what the proposed chains of causality are or how different activities should fit together. Furthermore, different actors might hold varied views on these relationships, and therefore part of the evaluation process should be to tease out how these various factors fit together. To date, two major approaches have been adopted in the evaluation of collaboration – theories of change (ToC) and realistic evaluation (RE). Table 3.2 outlines these approaches and their relative merits. It is important to note also that these approaches are not necessarily mutually exclusive, and some evaluation approaches have combined them, typically with a ToC approach embedded within RE (see, for example, Barnes et al, 1999; Secker et al, 2005). Despite both being theory-led, the approaches actually fulfil quite different roles, and complement each other in a number of ways.

The theory-based approaches outlined above contain differing functions for the evaluator: ToC is prospective with the evaluator involved in an iterative and ongoing process with those being evaluated (although, as Mason and Barnes, 2007, note, this has not always been the case in UK applications of this approach), while RE is retrospective and positions the evaluator in a much more 'traditional role' of outsider. Furthermore, one of the primary aims of ToC is to involve a wide variety of stakeholders within the evaluation process, which is usually less associated with RE. By locating ToC within an RE framework, it is possible gather multiple stakeholder theories, and from these to retrospectively identify the key configurations of contexts, mechanisms and outcomes. Indeed, these approaches strengthen each other through their differing conceptualisations of what constitutes 'theory' (Stame, 2004); ToC searches for 'grander' programme theories while RE tends to be much more concerned with a micro-psychological level of theory. Consolidating these two approaches allows the involvement of multiple stakeholders, fulfils a developmental function, overcomes issues of attribution and also identifies data relating to contexts, mechanisms and outcomes that may be of use in generalising knowledge across programmes. Therefore, when evaluating complex partnership initiatives, a consolidated ToC/RE approach is potentially more useful than either/or.

Although the rationale behind theory-based approaches is sensible, a number of attempts to apply these in practice have noted challenges with their applications (see, for example, Barnes et al, 2005; Dickinson, 2010). Moreover, the kinds of issues that theory-based approaches face tend to be the same sorts as those noted in Chapter 2 (for example, different stakeholder perspectives, unclear aspirations, lack of appropriate data etc). A key point here is that these kinds of approaches attempt to accommodate some of the complexities of collaborative working, although this does not necessarily render the evaluator any more equipped to overcome these issues. Perhaps the most powerful thing to note here is that there is an explicit acknowledgement of these issues, and this differentiates it from other approaches.

Table 3.2: Theory-led evaluation approaches

Approach	Brief description	Strengths	Limitations in practice	Example studies
Theories of Change (ToC)	A 'systematic and cumulative study of the links between activities, outcomes and contexts of the initiative' (Connell and Kubisch, 1998, p 18). This approach involves stakeholders surfacing the theories underpinning how and why a programme will work in as fine detail as possible, and identifying all the assumptions and sub-assumptions built into this process. ToC is concerned with theorising prospectively, rather than retrospectively (Connell and Kubisch, 1998), with the majority of surfacing exercises taking place during the planning stage of an initiative where there is an opportunity to explore a number of competing theories between stakeholders	By specifying what will happen in terms of short, medium and long-term outcomes of the interventions ToC seeks to overcome issues of attribution. Assists in the planning and implementation of an initiative. In-depth analysis of internal process issues. Multiple stakeholder involvement	External evaluation teams are rarely party to planning discussions in practice, so surfacing activities are unable to take place at this point (Sullivan et al, 2002). ToC suggests that all the theories and assumptions underpinning a programme can be surfaced, but in practice this can result in a number of differing realities being uncovered. ToC demands that one theory should prevail, but this is often not appropriate in practice. There are a number of practical difficulties in asking stakeholders to articulate such theories in the first place. Many find this an inherently difficult process	National evaluation of Health Action Zones (Barnes et al, 2005). National evaluation of LSPs (ODPM, 2005b)

(continued)

Table 3.2: Theory-led evaluation approaches (continued)

Realistic evaluation (RE)	RE suggests outcomes are characterised by the equation (C) Context + (M) Mechanism = (O) Outcome. Pawson and Tilley (1997) argue that no individual-level intervention works for everyone, and no institution-level intervention works everywhere. RE seeks to discover what mechanisms work for whom, and within which contexts	Overcomes issues of attribution by uncovering micro-level theory Identifies which mechanisms work for which individuals, and in which contexts Cumulative potential of knowledge with CMO configurations	Problems in identifying the outcomes of partnership working Problems in identifying mechanisms; Pawson and Tilley (1997) suggest these are often micro-level psychological processes, but they have often been interpreted as grander programmes or theories in practice Difficulties in conceptualising context (Dahler-Larsen, 2001; Calnan and Ferlie, 2003) Difficulties in differentiating mechanisms from context (Byng et al, 2005)	Evaluation of Health Education Authority's Integrated Purchasing Programme (Evans and Killoran, 2000)

Source: Dickinson (2006, p 379)

Helen Sullivan is an academic who has been involved in a number of large-scale evaluations of collaborative initiatives in the UK and internationally (including Health Actions Zones, LSPs and many more). In a 2011 paper she reflects on her experience and that of other evaluators in seeking the 'truth' demanded by the evidence-based movement over the late 1990s and first decade of the 2000s. She notes that 'despite the ambitions and opportunities presented by "theory-based evaluation", UK policy-makers (with the support of many evaluators) revised and refined theory-based approaches in order that they may be employed in the pursuit of "concrete factual realism"' (Sullivan, 2011, p 508). What Sullivan is highlighting here is that in the search for an objective and concrete version of reality that is generaliseable across a number of contexts, the search for 'truth' may have served to ignore the importance of the 'situated agency' of individuals and the room available to these actors to operate.

The concept of situated agency refers to the context in which individuals operate, and can refer to a range of different factors including culture, social processes, power and discourse. According to Sullivan, there may not be anything specific or concrete about collaborative working that we can apply across multiple contexts. The important point here may not be the availability of different sorts of evidence, but how actors use evidence and their ability to draw particular perspectives into processes of argumentation at a local level. What we should take from this argument is that if a crucial part of making collaboration work is the interaction of actors at a micro level and evaluations are not able to capture this, we may be missing part of an important picture about what makes partnerships work. The evidence about collaborative working may not be amenable to concrete factual realism, and it is important to consider precisely the types of mechanisms that evaluations might wish to focus on. This line of argument is considered in more detail below, in relation to the idea of performing collaboration.

In concluding this section we reiterate that the approach adopted in exploring collaboration will be determined through a range of different factors, such as the purpose of the evaluation, resources available and the nature of the collaboration being evaluated. There may be occasions when a large-scale quantitative approach is suitable, particularly when there is already a fairly well established evidence base demonstrating causal links. However, at other times intensive qualitative methods may be more useful in uncovering detailed perceptions of a range of stakeholders. It may be useful to return to the reasons for measuring performance discussed in Chapter 1, that were so clearly articulated by Behn (2003). As he notes, we need to be clear what our question is when we move to measuring – control, promote, learn, improve, motivate, budget or evaluate. Each demands a different perspective, different methodologies, and certainly different data. There are a series of questions (see Box 3.2) that you might want to ask yourself at the outset of an evaluation design, and the answers can help inform your choice of approach. Working through a systematic approach such as this will help provide transparency in your approach to the selection of evaluation design and also provide explicit acknowledgement of the limitations of any approach.

Box 3.2: Key questions to determine an evaluative approach

- What are the aims of the partnership you are evaluating?
- What are you aiming to evaluate, and why?
- What are you not aiming to evaluate, and why?
- What are the main stakeholder groups? What does each of these groups want the evaluation to deliver?
- Which of the stakeholder groups will be involved, to what degree, and why?
- What is the target group you are aiming to evaluate, and why?
- Who should conduct the evaluation?
- When should the evaluation start, and how long should it last?
- Are there any specific choices or constraints on the evaluation?
- What resources are available for the evaluation?

It may also be useful to consider:
- Are there any other similar evaluations that exist in the literature? What approach did they take? What challenges did they come up against? Do they make any specific suggestions about future research approaches?

What kinds of evidence about integration might we present to different groups?

Given the challenges we have set out about evaluating joint working, it is worthwhile considering multiple types of evidence, and how these might be presented to different groups. As we have set out to illustrate so far, different parties enter collaborative arrangements for different reasons, we measure performance to answer different questions, and these collaborations are often subject to external scrutiny. Further, service users and community groups may well demand evidence for the claims that are made about working together; this is especially so if it is intended to have a material impact on their lives. A prime minister will want different evidence to someone on the front line, a principle often referred to as the difference between 'shop floor' and 'top floor' informational needs.

Ultimately we need to think about the purpose of the evaluation and the question/s we are asking so we can gather appropriate evidence. Drawing again on Behn's reasons (see Box 1.2), we can think of some good examples:

- If we want to *promote* the achievements of the collaboration, we need to gather easily understood measures that can be interpreted by a broad audience of those whom we want to hear about our work. For example, being able to promote results such as fewer children in care as a result of a joint programme or more young people in jobs as a result of a joint programme can help to build support within partner organisations and more broadly. Presenting complex evaluation studies to these audiences often misses the mark as they tend to seek headline measures. These may be drawn from the more complex multifaceted evaluation, but to promote achievements, we need to look to different ways of getting the message across.

- If we want to *motivate* the parties to the collaboration, we will seek out very different evidence. Here we are looking to capture real-time data or useable feedback that allows us to learn, adapt, and which will drive real-time behavioural change in partners to the joint endeavour. Collecting data and analysing it in different ways, as discussed above, helps us to develop evidence. However, not all evidence is equal, according to the literature.

It should not be surprising that there is considerable debate around the very notion of evidence. This goes to fundamental questions of how we see the world, and whether there is some innate truth to be found within it. This also relates to methodological debates and revolves around questions such as the objective/subjective nature of evidence, the role of the researcher in that process, and the debate between quantitative and qualitative forms of data. Some scholars interested in evidence, and evidence-based policy, use the notion of a 'hierarchy of evidence' to rank the relative value or robustness of various types of evidence. From that they can discuss how rigorous the evidence is, and then make policy recommendations. A good example comes from a paper by Jensen and Lewis (2013) that offers counterviews on evidence-based policy, and compares the views of an economist (Jensen) and a political scientist (Lewis). In this paper, Jensen argues that not all evidence is of the same quality and therefore should not be treated equally. He discusses the hierarchy of evidence with the 'gold standard' of evidence providing 'robust causal evidence of the effects of a specific program' (p 4). In evaluating programmes, Jensen sets out a range of options (from lowest on the hierarchy to highest); evaluating economy-wide effects is, he argues, extraordinarily difficult. We adapt this somewhat to include our focus on more joined-up approaches (see Box 3.3).

Box 3.3 Various ways of evaluating programme effects on target groups

- Analyse a number of individuals before and after participation in the integrated programme. This approach is limited in that it cannot disentangle programme effects from other factors that may have had an impact on the outcome we observe. Select two *identical* individuals and observe their experience over time. This approach is limited because it is impossible to find two identical people, therefore making it difficult to disentangle the effects of the policy from the differences between the two people. Observe a treatment group (those that participate) and a control group (those that do not) before and after participation in the integrated programme. This approach is limited because we cannot separate out the effects from the programme from other factors that may have influenced the outcome.
- Observe the same individual in two different states of the world at the same time. The limitation is obvious – it is impossible to do this at the same time.
- Use a quasi-natural experiment where one group is subjected to an exogenous effect (that is, people do not choose to be in the group subjected to the effect) and another group is not. The limitation is that we have no control over who ends up in which group, and there will be many potential unobservable factors that influence outcomes. Allocate people randomly to a treatment group (those that participate in the integrated programme) or a control group (those that do not), and compare them over time. Some of the limitations include that we cannot 'trick' people into thinking they are getting the treatment as they would in a medical trial, and there are ethical and equity issues about adopting these randomised control trial (RCT) approaches.

Evaluation of policy, programmes and collaborations relies on a range of different types of evidence, but we would argue that most fits into the first and third categories above. There has been an increase in the use of RCTs because of arguments made about the robust and scientific evidence they can provide regarding 'what works'. Long used in medical research, RCTs have now been embraced by many in the social policy area as a means of testing a range of interventions and arrangements. They have become increasingly prominent in an era of austerity, where governments are keen to cut costs, and want to know more than ever whether programmes are actually working. Some departments have been using these in different ways for some time to generate evidence. For example, the Department for Work and Pensions has used RCTs to test whether additional support payments had an effect on getting people into work, and whether the intensity of signing on for welfare payments mattered (see Haynes et al, 2012, for many examples).

In a recent study, researchers used RCTs to test the efficacy of current approaches to preventing falls in hospitals, and provided evidence to show that some practices made no difference at all, and were taxing on staff time and resources (see Healy, 2016, for an overview). From our perspective, such approaches can also be used to test whether more joined-up interventions have an effect by designing RCTs that use different combinations of partners, for example, in new service design models.

Alongside this more 'scientific' approach to evidence has been the increased focus on 'big data' and the use of data analytics. As government organisations collect more and more data and allow access to it, and as our information-processing abilities improve, our ability to mine 'big data' and explore trends, patterns and broader effects may well improve. The big data phenomenon has many advocates who see this large-scale (usually quantitative) analysis as ground-breaking, not just in terms of undertaking more complex and systemic evaluation, but also in terms of designing interventions. More integrated datasets across government, for example, can allow for much more collaborative efforts between organisations and focus resources more effectively. Increasingly we will see more joined-up approaches designed around trends and patterns that are identified using data analytics.

An interesting international example comes from New Zealand, where the government claims to have transformed social welfare using a data analytics approach. The Ministry for Social Development started to do deep analysis of recipients and the spending that was focused on them from across government programmes. It could see that a small proportion of the population commanded a significant amount of its resources and efforts via various programmes. It developed a predictive risk model that allowed it to identify groups vulnerable to welfare dependency, and changed its approach to an investment approach to try to intervene early and prevent longer-term welfare dependency for these groups. Joined-up data, it argued, could be used to adopt more integrated approaches to social development that were focused on a small number of important results. Different stakeholders will have very different evidence demands. Some external scrutineers will seek detailed evaluations via, for example, cost-benefit analysis; others will seek headline results; and others will want evidence of the relationship and how the collaboration itself has performed. Users will have very different notions of how to show the collaboration is working for them (see some examples of outcomes users value in the next chapter). This can place significant demands on parties to the collaboration who may well see these numerous demands as burdensome.

An important part in the initial stages of developing the partnership, therefore, should be to seek clarity around these demands – often different partners will have various stakeholders with a range of evidence needs – and develop a plan for how to respond to these. Increasingly sharing data, and doing joint data collection, analysis and developing joint evaluation reports for multiple partners is to be encouraged, not least because it reduces the costs of evaluation for the parties to the collaboration. Working together to integrate data and to use approaches such as data analytics to identify common trends and co-design interventions can also help in underpinning joint work.

Performing governance: what is the additional work of collaboration?

Dickinson and Sullivan (2014) argue that one of the reasons why the collaboration literature has not been able to report much in the way of clear outcomes is because it typically treats collaboration as a rationalist and instrumental tool to bring about particular ends. More often these ends are goals such as improved service user outcomes or reduced inequalities in, for example, health, employment or education. Despite the fact that we lack evidence to demonstrate that this is the case, and there are plentiful accounts of the difficulties associated with collaborative practices and working arrangements, collaboration continues to be seen as a crucial activity for those involved in public services, and individuals and organisations invest significant time and resources in joint activities. Dickinson and Sullivan argue that this commitment to the idea of collaboration can be explained by taking a more complete view of collaboration. This involves taking into consideration the additional work of collaboration through the notion of cultural performance, which is associated with a quite different set of values and measures to those typically considered in the mainstream literature, and demonstrated through their social efficacy.

In setting out this argument, Dickinson and Sullivan draw on the work of Jon McKenzie (2001), who argues that performance is not a simple, coherent and stable concept; rather, it is dynamic – adaptive to and reflective of prevailing sociocultural and discursive forces. McKenzie identifies three different types of performance – organisational (efficiency), technological (effectiveness) and cultural (efficacy). The first two aspects are likely to be familiar to most and appear in the mainstream literature, and we have touched on many aspects of these so far in this book. Social efficacy is likely to be less familiar, although it broadly picks up on the themes we started to develop at the end of the first hot topic in this chapter. Social efficacy is about the constitution of meaning and affirmation of values achieved through an engagement with social norms – an aspect that new institutional theory also touches on, as illustrated in Chapter 1. Table 3.3. sets out these different aspects of performance in more detail.

Taking these ideas seriously means that we cannot simply look at the actions (and interactions) of individuals and organisations as being primarily motivated by rational drivers; their meaning goes beyond this. Decisions to collaborate are likewise complex, driven by motivations that are not rational, and many times not evidence-based, but reflective of particular values or meanings that are attached to collaboration itself.

Table 3.3: Three dimensions of performance

	Efficiency	Effectiveness	Efficacy
Paradigm	Performance management	Techno-performance. No specific paradigm, although closely aligned with computer science	Performance studies
Tools and techniques	Setting targets, performance indicators and measures, pay for performance, restructuring	Computers, statistical modelling, computer-aided design	Dramaturgy, reflexive practices, storytelling, ethnography
Performance is ...	Rational, it can be controlled for, predicted, managed, and ultimately delivered	Satisficing, different facets of performance are weighed up against one another. It is the result of a long and open series of negotiations and compromises	Always interactional in nature, it can both reaffirm existing traditions and beliefs or resist and adapt these

Source: Dickinson and Sullivan (2014, p 165)

Dickinson and Sullivan argue that exploring these motivations might help provide insights into why actors opt for, or persist with, collaboration in the face of limited evidence of its capacity to improve outcomes. They go on to argue that if we want to be able to evaluate the full impact of collaborative working, we need to ensure that we ask questions of all three dimensions of performance and not just efficiency and effectiveness, as the mainstream collaboration literature tends to do. This moves us beyond the types of evidence that are set out in Box

3.3, for example. To help in capturing this, they set out a framework populated by a set of questions that might be used to explore all three different dimensions of performance (see Table 3.4).

Table 3.4: A framework to explore the three dimensions of performance

Organisational efficiency	Technological effectiveness	Cultural efficacy
What different forms of collaboration exist, and how do their features differ from one another? Does collaboration lead to improved services? What measures demonstrate this? If collaboration does improve services and outcomes, which features of these collaborations produce these impacts? Is collaboration cost-effective compared to other forms of arrangements?	What types of technology are being used? To what degree do technologies manage to execute their prescribed tasks? What negotiations and compromises are made between possible technology performances?	What discourses of collaboration are present, and what performative work do discourses do? How is the performance of collaboration designed/ structured? How do actors perform a collaborative self? What are the affective dimensions of discourses and performances? What kinds of metaphors and symbols are present?

Source: Dickinson and Sullivan (2014, p 173)

Dickinson (2014) builds on the work of Dickinson and Sullivan (2014), and applies this framework to the evidence on collaborative working in three areas: child safeguarding, urban regeneration and the modernisation of health and social care. These areas were important sites of activity and investment under the New Labour governments, and Dickinson explores a more full account of collaborative working under these governments than has typically been presented in the mainstream literature. Traditional readings of this evidence base suggest that these different organisational arrangements had only a limited impact in practice. By incorporating a dimension of cultural efficacy into the process of evaluation, Dickinson identifies a series of further aspects of performance that have often been missed by the broader literature. This is an important observation, she argues, because the different dimensions of performance interact in interesting ways, which not only has implications for the overall impact of collaborative working, but also for the way in which we evaluate the success, or otherwise, of collaborations in practice.

As an example of this, the New Labour governments emphasised efficiency and effectiveness performances in the context of child safeguarding over successive terms. They introduced a set of reforms focusing on the structures of child safeguarding and systems concerning the sharing of information and data about children. Yet these reforms failed to take into consideration the practice of child safeguarding and the impact that this would have on practitioners at a local level. Many of these reforms did not fit with child safeguarding professionals' values and beliefs in terms of their roles, and as such, these reforms were resisted and subverted in parts. Where these were implemented and driven by the introduction of performance management techniques and measures, they are largely perceived to have had a detrimental impact on the ability of professionals to keep children safe. New forms of information-sharing technologies undermined the much more interpretive practices of child welfare professionals.

What we learn from this example is that it is not quite as easy to 'manage' issues of child safeguarding as it was perhaps sometimes presented, and that our traditional means of evaluation may not be telling us the full story on the relative success of more integrated approaches. For evaluators, the key point to recognise is that an important part of collaborative activity is what goes on within organisations, and how pursuit of this agenda has an impact on the identity and day-to-day practices of professionals and other key stakeholders. If we ignore these aspects, we miss the whole picture in terms of the impact of collaboration and the important interactions between different dimensions of performance.

Reflective exercises

1. Reflect on an evaluation of collaborative working you have been involved in or have read about. Do you think the most appropriate approach was chosen to evaluate this? Were there any difficulties reported by the evaluators? How might you overcome these? Do you think a different approach would have found different results?

2. Think of a collaborative endeavour that you think has been successful. Why do you think this (that is, what is 'success' to you)? What outcomes did it achieve? How might different stakeholders interpret these results? Did it have any negative effects?

3. Consider the different forms of evidence set out in this chapter. Which are most commonly used in your work setting? Why is that the case? What advantages might come from using different approaches?

4. Thinking about a collaboration you have been involved in, how integrated is the information that the partners draw on and the data they generate? What would a more sharing approach to data or a more 'big analytics'-focused approach allow you to do differently?

5. Imagine you have the opportunity to run an experiment in your area and you are asked to design a randomised control trial. What would you do? What would you focus on? What ethical issues might emerge?

6. Think about a collaboration you are a familiar with. Apply the questions from the cultural efficacy domain of Table 3.4. Do these tell you anything about the performance of that collaboration that you did not already know? How do you think these factors interact with other aspects of performance (for example, efficiency, effectiveness)?

Further reading and resources

This chapter has covered quite a broad area in terms of partnership evaluation, and readers may want to follow up specific studies or topics individually.

- For further information on the difference between theory-led and method-led evaluation see:
  - Pawson and Tilley's (1997) *Realistic evaluation*
  - Pawson's (2006) *Evidence-based policy* and (2013) *The science of evaluation: a realist manifesto*
  - Robson's (1993) *Real world research*
  - Chen's (1990) *Theory-driven evaluations*.
- The RAMESES Projects are funded by the National Institute of Health Research's Health Services and Delivery Research Programme, and aim to produce quality and publication standards and training materials for realist research approaches: www.ramesesproject.org
- For an interesting international example of the use of data analytics that provided integrated data for integrated approaches to social challenges, visit the New Zealand Ministry of Social Development: www.msd.govt.nz
- For a good overview on the potential for randomised control trials in policy, see Haynes et al's (2012) *Test, learn, adapt.*
- Dickinson's (2014) *Performing governance* sets out a more detailed version of issues relating to the additional impact of collaboration
- For those interested in cultural efficacy, McKenzie's (2001) *Perform or else* is a good place to start in the exploration of these ideas.

4

Useful frameworks and concepts

Drawing on the problems and the issues outlined in previous chapters, this chapter outlines a number of useful theoretical frameworks, tools and concepts to aid readers in understanding these issues in more depth, and to become better equipped to evaluate collaboration in health and social care. Although the complexities and challenges of evaluating collaborative working have been emphasised at a number of points throughout this text, in a number of ways evaluating collaborative working is no more challenging than other complex policy programmes or initiatives tend to be. In this respect, there are many resources available that may be drawn on when attempting to evaluate collaborative working. Those that seem to hold most salience for the context of health and social care have been outlined here, along with an indication of the conditions in which these will likely be most productive.

As we have also sought to reinforce throughout this text, one of the most important things to consider when seeking to evaluate collaborative working is to be clear about what you want to evaluate, what is of less importance, what resources you have available and within which timescales. If you are clear about these aspects from the start of the evaluation process, the likelihood is that you will be better equipped in approaching your project. The chapter finishes by setting out a framework that can help in identifying evaluation challenges and advice about how you might overcome these.

Classifying collaborations

If we are seeking to compare different collaborative working arrangements to one another, and we know that collaboration may take many different forms, it may be helpful to classify collaborative arrangements in some way. There are a variety of different frameworks and tools available to support this process, including those that focus on the degree of connection (see, for example, Keast et al, 2007, and their integration continuum); those that focus on the number of partners and the nature of their relationship (for example, Social Network Analysis, see Hinds and McGrath, 2006); and those that focus on different descriptions or models of collaboration (see, for example, Tompkinson, 2007's four categories of network, lead council, corporatist and supra-corporatist).

Some frameworks seek to combine several aspects at once, such as the depth versus breadth of relationship approach (Peck, 2002; Glasby, 2005) that encourages local health and social care collaborations to consider the balance they need to strike between depth (degree of interconnectedness) and breadth (number of partners) in order to achieve desired outcomes. Ling (2002) provides another example of an approach synthesising a number of these aspects, setting out four possible dimensions of collaboration covering factors such as the types of partnership members and who these are; what the nature of links between partners is; the scale of the collaboration and where its boundaries lie; and factors relevant to the organisational context.

We do not seek here to rehearse each of these different frameworks in detail, and will reserve more space for exploring some of the complex evaluative approaches in the remainder of the chapter. For those interested in exploring these issues in more detail, a helpful entry point is Granner and Sharpe's (2004) summary of measurement tools for coalition or partnership characteristics and functioning.

In Granner and Sharpe's review tools are organised into five general categories:

- member characteristics and perceptions;
- organisational or group characteristics;
- organisational or group processes and climate;
- general coalition function or scales bridging multiple constructs;
- impacts and outcomes.

A total of 59 different measures were identified. Since this time a range of other tools and approaches have been developed, although this is a good place to start for those new to the field. In doing so it is worth remembering that these have been developed from a range of different contexts, so if you are to use one of these, it is worth spending some time considering whether these will work in your specific context.

Process-based frameworks and measures

The bulk of tools that have been developed to date in the field of collaboration tend to fit within this category. Typically these identify specific factors or broad themes that are thought to be necessary for successful collaboration, and local areas assess their arrangements against these 'ideal scenarios'.

There are a number of different tools available, and these focus on more or less different aspects of collaborative working across differing contexts (Halliday et al, 2004). Examples include: the Partnership Assessment Tool (Hardy et al, 2003); the Working Partnership (Markwell et al, 2003); Partnership Readiness Framework (Greig and Poxton, 2001); the Victorian Health Promotion Foundation's Partnerships Analysis Tool (VicHealth, 2011); the Human Services Integration Measure (Browne et al, 2004); the Team Collaboration Assessment Rubric (Woodland and Hutton, 2012); and the Partnership Self-Assessment Tool (CACSH, 2010).

The introductory text in this series (Glasby and Dickinson, 2014) provides a review of some of these resources so we will not repeat that analysis here. What we will remind the reader of is that selecting a tool is an active choice, and you need to ensure that it fits both your purpose and context. This may mean using one of these available tools, or it may mean you want to think about adapting one of these to suit your specific situation (see Gomez-Bonnet and Thomas, 2015, for an example of this process).

Measuring outcomes

We have made the argument in this text that measuring the outcomes of collaborative working is far more of a challenge than it would initially appear. A key point to note here is that although we often assume that collaborations have clarity over what it is they are trying to deliver in terms of service user outcomes, experience suggests that this is often not the case. Without being sure about the outcomes you are trying to achieve, it can be difficult to set about measuring these in an effective way. Without a clear sense of what you are trying to achieve, there is a risk that evaluations end up using inappropriate outcome measures that do not necessarily link to the activity of that collaboration, or that they focus attention on inputs or processes to the detriment of outcomes. In this section we provide a very brief introduction to some of the many approaches and measures that exist within the broad literature, and it is worth spending time identifying precisely which kinds of measures you need and which will work best within the constraints of your evaluation.

In determining what outcomes you might want to measure, it is worth thinking about the different types of outcomes you are aiming to achieve. In a project in conjunction with the Social Care Institute for Excellence (SCIE), Glendinning et al (2006) identified which outcomes are important to older people (see Box 4.1). These are divided into change, maintenance and service process outcomes (as defined in Chapter 1), and different measures can be used in relation to the various aspects of outcomes.

Petch et al (2007) drew on this rubric in interviews with three different user groups – older people, people with a mental illness and people with learning difficulties. In Table 4.1 an overview is provided of what these different care groups described in terms of their aspired outcomes. Of course, in using these sorts of approaches, we need to be mindful of the fact that individuals often cross care groups, and may also have specific interests and values that go beyond those identified here. Therefore, if we are looking for a truly individualised sense of the outcomes that different service users value, we need to work with these individuals to understand them, and not simply rely on this sort of table.

Box 4.1: Outcomes that older people value

Outcomes involving change:
- Changes in symptoms or behaviours
- Improvements in physical functioning
- Improving morale

Outcomes involving maintenance or prevention:
- Meeting basic physical needs
- Ensuring personal safety and security
- Living in a clean and tidy environment
- Keeping alert and active
- Having control over everyday life

Service process outcomes:
- Feeing valued and being treated with respect
- Being treated as an individual
- Having 'a say' and control over services
- Value for money
- A 'good fit' with informal sources of support
- Compatibility with and respect for cultural and religious preferences

Source: Glendinning et al (2006)

One approach developed specifically for use in a collaborative setting to understand the full range of different stakeholder perspectives about the outcomes of collaborative working is POETQ (Jeffares and Dickinson, 2016). POETQ is an online tool designed to be engaging, comprehensive and methodologically robust. It is based on a Q methodology approach that asks participants to select from a range of statements, which they agree the most and least with, and then through a process of factor analysis identifies a series of viewpoints or 'worldviews' concerned with the impact that collaborative relationship is seeking to have.

POETQ has been used to investigate joint commissioning arrangements (among other collaborations) in recent years (Dickinson et al, 2013). Table 4.2 sets out five viewpoints identified through the research process relating to perspectives on what joint commissioning is set up to achieve. As Dickinson et al (2013) note, contrary to what we might be led to expect from the mainstream literature, these viewpoints cross different professional groups (that is, not all managers expressed an efficient perspective, just as all nurses did not express an ideal world perspective).

Within the outcomes literature there are a broad range of different measures that seek to quantify issues relating to aspects such as health status, mental health, functional ability, wellbeing and quality of life, among other factors. Here the aim is often to assess outcomes in an 'objective' and quantifiable way, so that comparisons can be made either between different initiatives or across time. In Box 4.2 a selection of different outcome indicators are presented, but these are just a few from a vast number in the literature. Like many of the more quantitative measures that we outline in this chapter, some have been empirically validated within particular contexts while others have not, and so it is worth doing some additional investigation before you embark on using any of these tools in practice. The evidence and data required to develop these indicators varies enormously.

Table 4.1: Outcomes across care groups

Outcome	Older people	Mental health	Learning disabilities
Quality of life			
Feeling safe	Knowing someone is there to keep an eye on the person = proactive monitoring Fear of crime in the neighbourhood Fear of falling	Knowing support is available should a crisis occur Fear of discrimination and stigma	Knowing there is someone trusted to talk to in case of crisis or distress Fear of harassment in the neighbourhood or from other service users
Having things to do	Getting out and about Availability of activities valued	Opportunities for employment and other meaningful activities	Choice of activities including physical and recreational Employment opportunities
Contact with other people	Social isolation is very common Home care is often the sole form of social contact Groups are valued by many (more often by females)	Social contact with other users is particularly valued Opportunities to socialise in a stigma-free environment are emphasised	Social contact with staff is particularly valued Social contact with other users is appreciated Establishing relationships in the community is challenging
Staying as well as you can be	Access to a range of professionals is often important in recovering from health crises Combating social isolation is important to sustain health	Access to support both preventatively and in the longer term if required, rather than restricted to crisis times	Role of staff in supporting access to mainstream and specialist health services

Table 4.1: Outcomes across care groups (continued)

Outcome	Older people	Mental health	Learning disabilities
Process			
Being listened to	Having a say in services	Having a say in services	Having a say in services
Feeling valued and treated with respect	Not being patronised Treated as an individual	Staff seeing beyond the label	Not being patronised
Having choices	Choice over timing of services and tasks undertaken Access to information about services	Choice over treatment options is important Choice of activities is appreciated Choice of accommodation is often restricted	Choice of activities is emphasised Choice over where people live and who with is important
Having people to rely on	Staff turning up and on time is often problematic, particularly in relation to home care Communication is important in such cases	Knowing that staff would turn up is important and a phone call to inform of changed arrangements is appreciated	Knowing that staff would turn up is important and a phone call to inform of changed arrangements is appreciated
Knowing someone will respond	Ability to contact someone and rely on a quick response in a crisis	Ability to contact someone and rely on a quick response in a crisis	Ability to contact someone and rely on a quick response in a crisis
Change			
Improving skills and confidence	Most older people using partnership services had experienced health crises and emphasised the role of services in restoring skills and confidence	Support with re-establishing skills and confidence following hospitalisation	Where periods of ill health had occurred, the role of services in restoring skills and confidence was valued

Table 4.1: Outcomes across care groups (continued)

Outcome	Older people	Mental health	Learning disabilities
Improving mobility	Restoring ability to walk where possible and/or supply adaptations where necessary	Support to use public transport	Availability of transport Support to use transport
Reducing symptoms	Reducing pain and discomfort Reducing symptoms of mental illness where required	Reducing and/or managing anxiety, depression and other aspects of mental illness	Reducing pain and discomfort Reducing symptoms of mental illness where required

Source: Miller (2012, p 27)

Table 4.2: Viewpoints of joint commissioning derived through a POETQ approach

Viewpoint	People outcomes	Partnership outcomes	Professional outcomes	Productivity outcomes
Ideal world commissioning	Joint commissioning produces better outcomes for service users	Joint commissioning leads to synergies between partners	There are differences between professional groups, but joint commissioning can help alleviate these	Joint commissioning can lead to better value for money
Efficient commissioning	Joint commissioning makes little difference in terms of service user outcomes	What joint commissioning symbolises is more important than what it does	Professionals having competing agendas can make joint working difficult	Joint commissioning is about making commissioning more efficient
Pluralist commissioning	Joint commissioning is about providing fairer access, inclusion and respect for service users	Joint commissioning can provide a holistic perspective, but doesn't necessarily deliver synergies	Differences between professionals have been overstated; joint commissioning offers an opportunity to dispel myths of 'us and them'	Joint commissioning is not about saving money
Personalised commissioning	The highest quality of service should be offered and service users should experience seamless services	Joint commissioning can help build empathy between professionals	Some professionals benefit more than others and joint commissioning can lead to buck-passing	Joint commissioning can be cumbersome and costly
Pragmatic commissioning	It is important to address the needs of 'real' people	Joint commissioning involves a lot of cost and effort	Joint commissioning can exacerbate the difficulties of joint working	Joint commissioning is good in theory, but in practice it is difficult to achieve and comes at a price

Source: Dickinson et al (2014, p 17)

Box 4.2: Examples of quantifiable outcome indicators

In measuring quality of life in health there are a wide range of different measures available, typically based on a series preference and measured on an interval scale. Some of the more popular include: the Standard Gamble, Time Trade-Off, Visual Analogue Scale and the Person Trade-Off technique (see Drummond et al, 2005).

The Camberwell Assessment of Need is a measurement tool that can be used to assess the degree to which the needs of an individual have been met over the preceding month across 22 health and social care domains (Phelan et al, 1995). Need can be assessed by either the service user or a professional, and the tool can be used to assess the degree to which the needs of an Individual are being met either at a specific point in time or across a time period.

There are a number of Health of the Nation Outcome Scales that are available for different groups, namely, Health of the Nation Outcome Scales for children and adolescents (HoNOSCA) for child and adolescent outcomes in mental health services; Health of the Nation Outcome Scales for older people (HoNOS 65+) for mental illness problems in older people; and HoNOS-secure, used with risk assessment measures in secure and forensic services. Each of these different scales contains a number of different items that are practitioner-rated and produce a score that can be used to assess how well service users are functioning (Speak et al, 2015).

The quality-adjusted life year (QALY) measure is a composite measure combining information on the length and quality of life. QALYs assign a health-related quality-of-life weight (a value) to each time period. A weight of 1 corresponds to optimal (or perfect) health, and 0 is a health state judged to be equivalent to death (Weinstein and Stason, 1977). Comparison can be made between different sorts of interventions on the basis of relative quality to outcome calculations.

The disability-adjusted life year (DALY) was first introduced by The World Bank to calculate the global burden of disease, and to be used as an outcome measure in cost-effectiveness analysis. It is a measure that combines the number of years lost due to premature death and the number of years lived with a disability. DALYs focus on disease and use a disease-specific description of health, whereas QALYs are more inclusive (Williams et al, 2012).

The Adult Social Care Outcomes Toolkit (ASCOT) is intended to capture information on an individual's social care-related quality of life (PSSRU, 2010). There are four different versions of this tool that vary in terms of length and who completes this (self-completion, staff, observation or a combination).

Comprehensive evaluation frameworks

Within the evaluation literature, a range of frameworks has been developed that seek to assess collaboration through a comprehensive framework (see, for example, Gajda, 2004; Koliba and Gajda, 2009; Thomson et al, 2009). The majority of these all-encompassing frameworks have been developed in the US to be relevant across a range of different policy fields. We highlight two here as examples of what approaches are available in the broader literature.

The Collaboration Evaluation and Improvement Framework (CEIF) builds on the research base to identify five entry points to aid thinking about when, where, and how to engage in evaluating collaboration (Woodland and Hutton, 2012). Figure 4.1 sets out an overview of this framework, which suggests the types of activities that might be considered in relation to different types of evaluative activities. Woodland and Hutton (2012) suggest a variety of different quantitative and qualitative data collection strategies appropriate to the different evaluation contexts at different stages of alliance development. This approach is intended to produce immediate findings about the collaboration in addition to data that can be used to help improve the quality of the relationships between partners.

The Collaboration Assessment Tool (CAT) was developed from a study by Mattessich and Monsey (1992) analysing effective collaboration practices. This study has since been further developed into a framework

Figure 4.1: Collaboration Evaluation and Improvement Framework

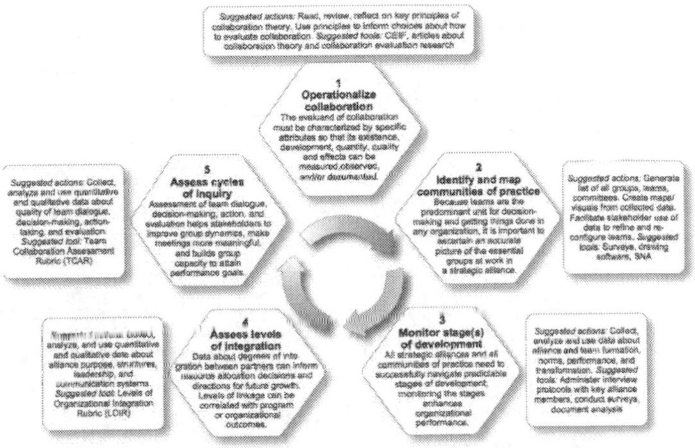

Source: Rebecca H. Woodland, Michael S. Hutton, 'Evaluating organizational collaborations: suggested entry points and strategies', *American Journal of Evaluation* (33, 3), Copyright © 2012. Reprinted by permission of SAGE Publications Inc

of 20 factors organised into six categories, which have subsequently been developed by Marek et al (2014) into a more theoretical approach with seven factors that have been identified as critical for effective collaboration: context, members, process and organisation, communication, function, resources, and leadership. Across the seven factors, a CAT survey was developed with 69 different items that participants are asked to self-rate on a Likert-type scale from 1-5 (where 1 is strongly disagree and 5 strongly agree). CAT can be used 'both as an informal inventory and a validated tool to evaluate the current functioning of coalitions. Employing this tool can help coalitions better understand their strengths and weaknesses in working collaboratively, leading to more successful outcomes' (Marek et al, 2014, p 11).

Better evaluation of collaboration

In this final section we summarise what some of the key lessons are in terms of the effective evaluation of collaborative working. Although evaluating collaboration is often difficult and complex, it is no more so than the majority of other large public sector initiatives that are evaluated on a daily basis. Indeed, it is difficult to think of any large-scale public sector initiative that simply involves one organisation and does not draw – at least in part – from other sectors, industries, agencies or individuals. This is a reflection of the nature of the world we live in, and a trend that looks ever more likely to grow rather than retreat, and this at least partly explains the recent growth in this literature. As such, we may usefully draw lessons from other large-scale evaluations about how we might go about evaluating partnerships.

One such source that we draw on here is the Making the Shift project that sought to learn from a series of pilot sites that were shifting care from hospitals into the community (Ham et al, 2007). Clearly there is an inter-agency aspect to these pilot projects, even if this is not their specific focus. While many of the lessons learned were to do with the design, organisation and management of the pilots, a key issue was around measuring and monitoring progress. In particular:

- Some areas found it difficult to develop ways to measure their success because they had not fully defined the scope of their projects.
- Some project teams felt they had insufficient experience to consider the range of measurement strategies possible, including knowledge of existing datasets or expertise to develop questionnaires.
- Some projects felt that they had inadequate capacity to process or analyse any data emerging from their projects.

In response, the evaluation found that there were three important questions to keep in mind throughout the development and subsequent evaluation of pilot projects:

1 What is the project designed to achieve? (in particular, any numerical targets)
2 What is the situation now? (baseline data, sources and person responsible for compiling)
3 How will we know if we have made a difference? (follow-up sources, comparators and person responsible)

While each pilot adopted different approaches, there were three key areas that were important to measure in most projects:

- changes in service use/resource use (such as emergency admission rates);
- financial changes/cost-benefit analyses;
- service users' experience and satisfaction.

The experience of the pilots also helped to identify a series of key principles to keep in mind when devising ways of measuring progress (see Box 4.3). Basic though these messages appear, a key recommendation from those actively involved in trying to shift care out of hospitals was to *keep any evaluation mechanism simple and practical*, building on existing data and structures wherever possible. Tracking progress is also important because we can learn much on the journey towards a goal that can inform our practice. Recent work by Shelley Metzenbaum (see the 'Further reading' section at the end of this chapter), who led the Obama administration's performance agenda in the US, focuses on the principle of progress and the importance of clear goals. She also stresses that we should be able to explain our progress towards goals, even when they are not met.

Thinking back to an earlier chapter, we outlined a number of the key challenges that evaluations of collaborative working tend to encounter. Drawing on the various evaluations, frameworks and theories discussed up to this point, this chapter concludes by offering a table that lists these key challenges, the questions evaluators might wish to ask, and the tools available to overcome these issues (see Table 4.3).

Box 4.3: Key evaluation principles from the Making the Shift project

1. Focus on simple methods that will not take too much time to collect or analyse.
2. Focus on three to five key indicators per project, rather than long lists of potential metrics.
3. Focus on routinely collected data where possible, rather than developing new datasets.
4. There must be some comparator in order to demonstrate a shift (either before and after or comparison sites).
5. Every stated project objective must have an associated measure.
6. Involve information analysts and other appropriate staff from the project outset.
7. Set realistic timeframes for collating data and assign people with specific responsibility for this.
8. Finding out what does not work is as important as whether or not there is a measurable change.
9. Some measures need to be ongoing to provide scope for examining change over time.
10. It is possible to draw on external support to assist with measurement and metrics, or to provide training for managers and front-line staff.

Source: Ham et al (2007, p 34)

Table 4.3: Evaluation challenges and how these may be overcome

Evaluation challenge	Questions you might ask to overcome this and available tools
Should I measure process, outcome or both?	What is it that the collaboration is aiming to achieve and you want to find out through the evaluation? If you want to look at how well partners are working together, use a 'health assessment' toolkit. If you are interested in outcomes, select an appropriate outcome indicator. However, if the collaboration is particularly complex or causal links between activities and outcomes are weak, you may need to evaluate both process and outcome
Which outcome measures?	Be clear about what it is that you are setting out to measure from the outset. Ascertaining whether there is clarity over outcomes could be established through a ToC approach or the use of POETQ. What outcome indicators are already collected? Can they be used? Check with service users which outcomes they value (Glendinning et al's 2006 framework may be useful here)
Multiple definitions of collaborations – how can you generalise lessons?	What aspect or feature of collaboration are you attempting to evaluate? Which other collaborations demonstrate similar features? It may be useful to classify collaborations here using one of the approaches in Granner and Sharpe (2004)
Incorporating multiple perspectives	Select a methodology that allows many stakeholders to speak
Context	Map out all the factors within the local context that you think may have an impact on the functioning of the collaboration. You may want to do this by yourself, with a group of key stakeholders, or form this through identification of key themes from interviews/focus groups/documentary analysis
Attribution	Look at previous literature to establish whether there is any evidence relating to causal relationships between key factors that you have identified. If such links are well established you may be able to presume attribution using a comparative or quasi-experimental evaluation design (controlling for contextual factors). If there is no such evidence base you may want to consider using a theory-led evaluation approach to overcome this difficulty

Table 4.3: Evaluation challenges and how these may be overcome (continued)

Evaluation challenge	Questions you might ask to overcome this and available tools
Unintended consequences?	Particularly within complex open systems it is difficult to capture any additional knock-on or unintended consequences that partnerships might produce. By speaking to local stakeholders who are in tune with the local context, you may be able to identify any additional impacts that have been felt. This will normally involve drawing on a wider range of stakeholders than simply the core group who would normally be involved in such an evaluation
Outcome timescales	When would you expect to see changes in outcomes? Map these out in terms of outputs, immediate, intermediate and long-term outcomes and be transparent about this
How can you prove you have prevented something? (the counterfactual challenge)	In the national evaluation of intermediate care (Barton et al, 2006), staff admitting patients to intermediate care were asked to consider what would have happened to the patient had the scheme not been in place. Charting hypothetical baselines may be a useful way of demonstrating what could have happened if the partnership had not been introduced

Reflective exercises

1. Obtain one of the classification tools outlined in this chapter, and apply it to a number of different types of collaborations that you are familiar with or have read about. What does this tell you about that relationship, and is this helpful?

2. Obtain one of the process assessment tools outlined in this chapter, and apply it to a number of different types of collaborations that you are familiar with or have read about. What does this tell you about that relationship, and is this helpful?

3. Reflect on a partnership you know or have read about. Construct all the theories of change (ToC) you can think of concerning what this partnership is aiming to achieve in terms of service user outcomes. If you can, get a friend or a colleague to carry out the same exercise. How do your ToC compare?

4. Read about one or more outcome measures and think about how applicable it would be to a collaboration you are familiar with. What would this tell you about the impact of this working relationship and what would it miss?

Further reading and resources

Most of the key texts and resources for this chapter are summarised in the relevant sections for readers to explore in more detail.

- Useful websites to aid this search include:
  - Social Care Institute for Excellence (SCIE): www.scie.org.uk
  - Social Policy Research Unit (SPRU): www.york.ac.uk/inst/spru/
  - Personal Social Services Research Unit (PSSRU): www.pssru.ac.uk/
  - See the IBM Center for the Business of Government profile page for Dr Shelley Metzenbaum, which includes links to a range of reports she has prepared on performance: www. businessofgovernment.org/bio/shelley-h-metzenbaum
- Further details on selected tools and approaches can be found at the sources indicated below:

- Team – Collaboration Assessment Rubric (TCAR): www. nsfepscor2015.org/uploads/3/9/6/3/39630685/team_ collaboration_assessment_rubric.pdf
- Collective Impact Framework: www.collaborationforimpact.com/ collective-impact/
- Adult Social Care Outcomes Toolkit (ASCOT): www.pssru.ac.uk/ ascot/
- Granner and Sharpe's coalition measurement review: http:// prevention.sph.sc.edu/tools/CoalitionEvalInvent.pdf

- Williams et al's (2012) *Rationing in health care* sets out an overview of a number of different economic evaluation tools.
- Miller's (2012) *Individual outcomes* provides an insightful overview into the processes of defining individuals service user outcomes in Scotland.

5

Recommendations for policy and practice

Drawing on the questions, summaries and frameworks set out in this book, there are a series of practical recommendations and potential warnings that arise, for both policy and practice.

For policy-makers

- Given that collaboration takes so many different forms and is driven by different goals, they cannot be expected to deliver the same outcomes. More research is required to establish *what kinds of collaborative arrangements can produce which kinds of outcomes, for which kinds of service users, when, and how?*
- Central government needs to be clearer about what it reasonably expects collaborative working to deliver, and under which circumstances collaborations are appropriate and, importantly, when they are not.
- Political timescales and evaluation timescales are often incompatible. When commissioning evaluations of collaborative working, this needs to be carefully considered.
- Service users are not homogeneous groups, and individuals (particularly those with complex or challenging needs) require specific support. More closely involving individuals in determining the nature of their own care may produce positive impacts, in terms of both service effectiveness and efficiency. This can produce different ways of joining up services and empowering individuals to achieve better outcomes, and is worthy of further exploration of its usefulness beyond social care. It can also create new demands for evidence of performance.

- Although various structural, legal and technical fixes have aided the formation of health and social care partnerships to a certain extent, what local organisations and front-line services also need is more detail on how they might actually go about producing better collaborative working, and what this would entail. We need to be attuned to the fact that collaboration has impacts across a range of different dimensions, and if we do not take this into consideration, there may be unanticipated consequences.
- Although a partnership may be useful in producing some kinds of outcomes for some kinds of service users, it is not a panacea or a solution to all difficulties. If this concept continues to be used incessantly without appropriate research evidence to back it up, it risks losing legitimacy. Think more carefully about how and when this concept should be invoked.

For local organisations and front-line services

- Collaboration is not the answer to every difficulty. Think long and hard about why you need to establish a partnership, and what outcomes you hope to achieve for service users.
- Having a focus on what outcomes it is that you are aiming to achieve for service users is often helpful in working through debates over how services should be delivered. Once the function of a collaboration has been established and agreed on between partners, it is then possible to work through the form that services will take. Establishing form before function can potentially be damaging.
- Be clear about what the purposes of the collaborative arrangement are, why it is you are undertaking an evaluation, and what you hope to achieve by it before you start out.
- Carefully consider which stakeholders need to be involved in any evaluation, and be clear about why it is you are not involving others.
- Build periodic evaluation into any collaborative endeavour. Continually revisit the issue of outcomes, checking whether the desired aims of the partnership are still the same, and whether the form is appropriate in seeking to achieve these aims.

It is difficult to be definitive about collaboration. As this text – and indeed, the rest of this series – highlights, collaboration is a tricky thing to make work at the best of times. Currently collaboration is somewhat in vogue within national and international public policy and more widely within the commercial sector. In one sense this is a positive achievement, and more attention than ever has been focused on attempting to provide seamless and accessible services to individuals, families and communities who are often in times of need or experiencing chronic and complex problems.

However, collaborative working offers enormous challenges in terms of the ways in which individuals, organisations and sectors can work together in productive and creative ways. The current popularity of this concept has also meant that many different ways of working have been subsumed under one umbrella concept, when, in fact, collaboration takes many forms and is propelled by a range of different drivers. This, in turn, poses an enormous evaluative challenge. The continuation of the invocation of the collaboration concept is ultimately dependent on an ability to clearly evidence this way of working. Without demonstrating the positive – and not so positive – impacts that collaboration has, we risk undermining its value.

Implicit in assumptions about collaboration is that it is necessarily a 'good thing', and to some degree it may well be. However, to keep on expecting front-line staff to engage with this agenda when their everyday experiences are of challenging behaviours and organisational and procedural complexity, while wider research is unable to say little definitive about benefits, is naive.

It is imperative that more is invested in research so we are better able to say what types of benefits collaboration is able to deliver for whom; how local organisations can work together more effectively to produce better collaborative working; and, importantly, when collaboration is not necessary and might even be counter-productive. Such information would reinvigorate the collaboration agenda and renew its legitimacy.

References

6, P., Goodwin, N., Peck, E. and Freeman, T. (2006) *Managing networks of twenty-first century organisations*, Basingstoke: Palgrave.

6, P., Leat, D., Seltzer, K. and Stoker, G. (2002) *Towards holistic governance: The new reform agenda*, Basingstoke: Palgrave.

Alford, J. (2009) *Engaging public sector clients: From service-delivery to co-production*, Basingstoke: Palgrave Macmillan.

Alford, J. and O'Flynn, J. (2012) *Rethinking public service delivery: Managing with external providers*, Basingstoke: Palgrave Macmillan.

Alter, C. and Hage, J. (1993) *Organizations working together*, Newbury Park, CA: Sage Publications.

Andrews, R. and Entwistle, T. (2010) 'Does cross-sectoral partnership deliver? An empirical exploration of public service effectiveness, efficiency and equity', *Journal of Public Administration Research and Theory*, vol 20, no 3, pp 679-701.

Asthana, S., Richardson, S. and Halliday, J. (2003) 'Partnership working in public policy provision: a framework for evaluation', *Social Policy & Administration*, vol 36, pp 780-95.

Audit Commission (2005) *Governing partnerships: Bridging the accountability gap*, London: Audit Commission.

Axford, N. and Berry, V. (2005) 'Measuring outcomes in the "new" children's services', *Journal of Integrated Care*, vol 13, pp 12-23.

Balloch, S. and Taylor, M. (2001) *Partnership working: Policy and practice*, Bristol: Policy Press.

Banks, G. (2009) *Evidence-based policy making: What is it? How do we get it?*, Canberra, ACT: Commonwealth of Australia.

Banks, P. (2002) *Partnerships under pressure: A commentary on progress in partnership working between the NHS and local government*, London: The King's Fund.

Barnes, M., Bauld, L., Benezeval, M., Judge, K., Killoran, A., Robinson, R. and Wigglesworth, R. (1999) *Health Action Zones: Learning to make a difference*, Canterbury: University of Kent.

Barnes, M., Bauld, L., Benezeval, M., Judge, K., Mackenzie, M. and Sullivan, H. (2005) *Health Action Zones: Partnerships for health equity*, London: Routledge.

Barrett, G., Sellman, D. and Thomas, J. (2005) *Interprofessional working in health and social care: Professional perspectives*, Basingstoke: Palgrave.

Barton, P., Bryan, S., Glasby, J., Hewirr, G., Jagger, C., Kaambwa, B. et al (2006) *A national evaluation of the costs and outcomes of intermediate care for older people*, Birmingham and Leicester: Health Services Management Centre and Leicester Nuffield Research Unit.

Behn, R.D. (2003) 'Why measure performance? Different purposes require different measures', *Public Administration Review*, vol 63, no 5, pp 586-606.

Birckmayer, J.D. and Weiss, C.H. (2000) 'Theory-based evaluation in practice. What do we learn?', *Evaluation Review*, vol 24, pp 407-31.

Browne, G., Roberts, J., Gafni, A., Byrne, C., Kertyzia, J. and Loney, P. (2004) 'Conceptualizing and validating the Human Services Integration Measure', *International Journal of Integrated Care*, vol 4, April-June, pp 1-9.

Butler, I. and Drakeford, M. (2005) *Scandal, social policy and social welfare*, Bristol: Policy Press.

CACSH (Center for the Advancement of Collaborative Strategies in Health) (2010) *Partnership Self-Assessment Tool: Questionnaire*, New York: CACSH (www.nccmt.ca/about/partnerships).

Challis, L., Fuller, S., Henwood, M., Klein, R., Plowden, W., Webb, A., Whittingham, P. and Wistow, G. (1988) *Joint approaches to social policy: Rationality and practice*, Cambridge: Cambridge University Press.

Chen, H.-T. (1990) *Theory-driven evaluations*, London: Sage Publications.

Cresswell, J.W. (2014) *Research design: Qualitative, quantitative and mixed methods approaches* (4th edn), London: Sage.

Curry, N. and Ham, C. (2010) *Clinical and service integration: The route to improved outcomes*, London: The King's Fund.

Davies, P.T. (2000) 'Contributions from qualitative research', in H. Davies, S. Nutley and P. Smith (eds) *What works? Evidence-based policy and practice in public services*, Bristol: Policy Press, pp 291-316.

de Bruijn, H. (2002) *Managing performance in the public sector*, London: Routledge.

DCLG (Department for Communities and Local Government) (2014) *National evaluation of the Troubled Families programme*, London: The Stationery Office (www.gov.uk/government/publications/national-evaluation-of-the-troubled-families-programme).

DfT (Department for Transport) (2005) *Evaluation of local strategic partnerships: Interim report*, London: Office of the Deputy Prime Minister.

DH (Department of Health) (1969) *Committee of Enquiry into allegations of ill-treatment of patients and other irregularities at the Ely Hospital, Cardiff*, Cmnd 3975, London: HMSO.

DH (1998) *Partnership in action: New opportunities for joint working between health and social services*, London: DH.

DH (2006) *Our health, our care our say: A new direction for community services*, London: The Stationery Office.

DH (2013) *Integrated care: Our shared commitment*, London: DH.

Dickinson, H. (2010) 'The importance of being efficacious: English health and social care partnerships and service user outcomes', PhD thesis, University of Birmingham.

Dickinson, H. (2014) *Performing governance: Partnerships, culture and New Labour*, Basingstoke: Palgrave Macmillan.

Dickinson, H. and Carey, G. (2016) *Managing and leading in interagency settings* (2nd edn), Better Partnership Working series, Bristol: Policy Press.

Dickinson, H. and Glasby, J. (2010) 'Why partnership working doesn't work', *Public Management Review*, vol 12, pp 811-28.

Dickinson, H. and Sullivan, H. (2014) 'Towards a general theory of collaborative performance: The importance of efficacy and agency', *Public Administration*, vol 92, no 1, pp 161-77.

Dickinson, H., Glasby, J., Nicholds, A., Jeffares, S., Robinson, S. and Sullivan, H. (2013) *Joint commissioning in health and social care: An exploration of definitions, processes, services and outcomes, Final report*, Southampton: National Institute for Health Research (NIHR) Services Delivery and Organisation Programme.

DiMaggio, P.J. and Powell, W.W. (1991) *The new institutionalism in organizational analysis*, London: University of Chicago Press.

Drummond, M.F., Schulpher, M.J., Torrance, G.W, O'Brien, B.J. and Stoddart, G.L. (2005) *Methods for economic evaluation of health care programmes* (3rd edn), Oxford: Oxford University Press.

Dunleavy, P. (1991) *Democracy, bureaucracy and public choice*, Hemel Hempstead: Harvester Wheatsheaf.

Dunt, I. (2015) 'The government is silencing its own drug experts', 19 June (www.politics.co.uk/blogs/2015/06/19/the-government-is-silencing-its-own-drug-experts).

Edwards, A., Barnes, M., Plewis, I. et al (2006) *Working to prevent the social exclusion of children and young people: Final lessons from the national evaluation of the Children's Fund*, Birmingham and London: University of Birmingham and Department for Education and Skills.

Emerson, R.M. (1962) 'Power dependence relations', *American Sociological Review*, vol 27, pp 31-40.

Entwistle, T. (2014) *Collaboration and public services improvement. Evidence review prepared for the Commission on Public Service Government and Delivery*, PPIW Report No 2, Cardiff: Public Policy Institute for Wales.

Gajda, R. (2004) 'Utilizing collaboration theory to evaluate strategic alliances', *American Journal of Evaluation*, vol 25, no 1, pp 65-77.

Glasby, J. (2005) 'The integration dilemma: how deep and how broad to go?', *Journal of Integrated Care*, vol 13, no 5, pp 27-30.

Glasby, J. and Beresford, P. (2006) 'Who knows best? Evidence-based practice and the service user contribution', *Critical Social Policy*, vol 26, no 1, pp 268-84.

Glasby, J. and Dickinson, H. (2014) *Partnership working in health and social care: What is integrated care and how can we deliver it?* (2nd edn), Better Partnership Working series, Bristol: Policy Press.

Glendinning, C., Hudson, B., Hardy, B. and Young, R. (2002) *National evaluation of notifications for the use of the Section 31 partnership flexibilities in the Health Act 1999: Final project report*, Leeds and Manchester: Nuffield Institute for Health and National Primary Care Research and Development Centre.

Glendinning, C., Clarke, S., Hare, P., Kotchetkova, I., Maddison, J. and Newbronner, L. (2006) *Outcomes-focused services for older people*, London: Social Care Institute for Excellence.

Gomez-Bonnet, F. and Thomas, M. (2015) 'A three-way approach to evaluating partnerships: Partnership survey, integration measure and social network analysis', *Evaluation Journal of Australia*, vol 15, no 1, pp 28-37.

Granner, M.L. and Sharpe, P.A. (2004) 'Evaluating community coalition characteristics and functioning: a summary of measurement tools', *Health Education Research*, vol 19, pp 514-32.

Gray, J. (1997) *Evidence-based health care: How to make health policy and management decisions*, London: Churchill Livingstone.

Greener, I. (2015) 'Wolves and big yellow taxis: How would be known if the NHS is at death's door?', *International Journal of Health Policy Management*, vol 4, no 10, pp 687-9.

Greig, R. and Poxton, R. (2001) 'From joint commissioning to partnership working – will the new policy framework make a difference?', *Managing Community Care*, vol 9, no 4, pp 32-8.

Halliday, J., Asthana, S.N.M. and Richardson, S. (2004) 'Evaluating partnership: the role of formal assessment tools', *Evaluation*, vol 10, pp 285-303.

Ham, C. (1977) 'Power, patients and pluralism', in K. Barnard and K. Lee (eds) *Conflicts in the NHS*, London: Croom Helm. Ham, C., Parker, H., Singh, D. and Wade, E. (2007) *Final report on the Care Closer to Home: Making the Shift programme*, Warwick: NHS Institute for Innovation and Improvement.

Hardy, B., Hudson, B. and Waddington, E. (2003) *Assessing strategic partnership: The Partnership Assessment Tool*, London: Office of the Deputy Prime Minister and Nuffield Institute for Health.

Harrison, S. (1999) 'Clinical autonomy and health policy: past and futures', in M. Exworthy and S. Halford (eds) *Professionals and the new managerialism in the public sector*, Buckingham: Open University Press, pp 50-64.Hayes, S.L., Mann, M.K., Morgan, F.M. and Weightman, A. (2011) 'Collaboration between local health and local government agencies for health improvement', *Cochrane Database of Systematic Reviews*, vol 10, no 6, June.

Haynes, L., Service, O., Goldacre, B. and Torgerson, D. (2012) *Test, learn, adapt: Developing public policy with randomised control trials*, London: Behavioural Insights Team, Cabinet Office (www.gov.uk/ government/uploads/system/uploads/attachment_data/file/62529/ TLA-1906126.pdf).

Haynes, P. (2015) *Managing complexity in the public services* (2nd edn), London: Routledge.

Head, B.W. (2014) 'Public administration and the promise of evidence-based policy: experience in and beyond Australia', *Asia Pacific Journal of Public Administration*, vol 36, no 1, pp 48-59.

Head, B.W. and O'Flynn, J. (2015) 'Australia: Building policy capacity for managing wicked policy problems', in A. Massey and K. Johnston (eds) *The international handbook of public administration and governance*, Cheltenham: Edward Elgar, pp 341-68.

Healy, F. (2016) 'Editorial: Preventing falls in hospitals', *British Medical Journal*, vol 352, i251.

Himmelman, A.T. (1996) 'On the theory and practice of transformational collaboration: from social service to social justice', in C. Huxham (ed) *Creating collaborative advantage*, London: Sage Publications, 19-43.Himmelman, A.T. (2001) 'On coalitions and the transformation of power relations: collaborative betterment and collaborative empowerment', *American Journal of Community Psychology*, vol 29, pp 277-84.

Hinds, P. and McGrath, C. (2006) 'Structures that work: social structure, work structure, and performance in geographically distributed teams', Proceedings of the Conference on 'Computer supported cooperative work', Banff, Alberta.

HM Treasury (2003) *Every Child Matters*, London: The Stationery Office.

Hood, C. (1991) 'A public management for all seasons', *Public Administration*, vol 69, pp 3-19.

Hudson, B. (2000) 'Inter-agency collaboration: a sceptical view', in A. Brechin, H. Brown and M. Eby (eds) *Critical practice in health and social care*, Milton Keynes: Open University Press.

Hudson, B., Exworthy, M., Peckham, S. and Callaghan, G. (1999) *Locality partnerships: The early primary care group experience*, Leeds: Nuffield Institute for Health.

Hughes, J. and Weiss, J. (2007) 'Simple rules for making alliances work', *Harvard Business Review*, 14 November, pp 1-10.

Huxham, C. (ed) (1996) *Creating collaborative advantage*, London: Sage.

Huxham, C. and Hibbert, P. (2008) 'Hit or myth? Stories of collaborative success', in J. O'Flynn and J. Wanna (eds) *Collaborative governance? A new era of public policy in Australia?*, Canberra, ACT: ANU Press, pp 45-50.

Huxham, C. and Vangen, S. (2004) 'Doing things collaboratively: Realizing the advantage or succumbing to inertia', *Organizational Dynamics*, vol 33, no 2, pp 190-201.

Jeffares, S. and Dickinson, H. (2016) 'Evaluating collaboration: The creation of an online tool employing Q methodology', *Evaluation*, vol 22, no 1, pp 91-107.

Jelphs, K., Dickinson, H. and Miller, R. (2016) *Working in teams* (2nd edn), Better Partnership Working series, Bristol: Policy Press.

Jensen, P. and Lewis, J.M. (2013) *Evidence-based policy: Two countervailing views*, Issues Paper Series no 1/2013, Melbourne, VIC: Melbourne School of Government, University of Melbourne.

Jupp, B. (2000) *Working together: Creating a better environment for cross-sector partnerships*, London: Demos.

Kanter, R.M. (1994) 'Collaborative advantage: the art of alliances', *Harvard Business Review*, vol 72, pp 96-108.

Keast, R., Brown, K. and Mandell, M. (2007) 'Getting the right mix: unpacking integration meanings and strategies', *International Public Management Journal*, vol 10, no 1, pp 9-33.

Kirk, J. and Miller, M. (1986) *Reliability and validity in qualitative research*, London: Sage Publications.

Klein, R. (2000) *The new politics of the NHS*, London: Longman.

Koliba, C. and Gajda, R. (2009) 'Communities of practice as an analytical construct: Implications for theory and practice', *International Journal of Public Administration*, vol 32, pp 97-135.

Laming, H. (2003) *The Victoria Climbié Inquiry: Report of an inquiry*, London: The Stationery Office.

Laming, W. (2009) *The protection of children in England: A progress report*, London: The Stationery Office.

Lazenbatt, A. (2002) *The evaluation handbook for health professionals*, London: Routledge.

Leathard, A. (ed) (1994) *Going inter-professional: Working together for health and welfare*, Hove: Routledge.

Leutz, W. (1999) 'Five laws for integrating medical and social services: lessons from the United States and the United Kingdom', *The Milbank Quarterly*, vol 77, no 1, pp 77-110.

Levine, S. and White, P.E. (1962) 'Exchange as a conceptual framework for the study of interorganizational relationships', *Administrative Science Quarterly*, vol 5, pp 583-601.

Lewis, M. and Hartley, J. (2001) 'Evolving forms of quality management in local government: lessons from the Best Value pilot programme', *Policy & Politics*, vol 29, pp 477-96.

Ling, T. (2002) 'Delivering joined-up government in the UK: dimensions, issues and problems', *Public Administration*, vol 80, pp 615-42.

Lundin, M. (2007) 'When does cooperation improve public policy implementation?', *The Policy Studies Journal*, vol 35, no 4, pp 629-52.

Marek, L.I., Brock, D.P. and Savla, J. (2014) 'Evaluating collaboration for effectiveness: Conceptualization and measurement', *American Journal of Evaluation*, pp 1-19.

Markwell, S., Watson, J., Speller, V., Platt, S. and Younger, T. (2003) *The working partnership*, London: Health Development Agency.

Mason, A., Goddard, M., Weatherly, H. and Chalkley, M. (2015) 'Integrating funds for health and social care: an evidence review', *Journal of Health Services Research & Policy*, vol 20, no 3, pp 177-88.

Mason, P. and Barnes, M. (2007) 'Constructing theories of change: methods and sources', *Evaluation*, vol 13, pp 151-70.

Mattessich, P.W. and Monsey, B.R. (1992) *Collaboration: What makes it work?*, Saint Paul, MN: Amherst H. Wilder Foundation.

McCray, J. and Ward, C. (2003) 'Editorial notes for November: leading interagency collaboration', *Journal of Nursing Management*, vol 11, pp 361-3.

McKenzie, J. (2001) *Perform or else: From discipline to performance*, London: Routledge.

McLaughlin, H. (2004) 'Partnerships: panacea or pretence?', *Journal of Interprofessional Care*, vol 18, pp 103-13.

McNulty, T. and Ferlie, E. (2002) *Re-engineering health care: The complexities of organizational transformation*, Oxford: Oxford University Press.

Miller, E. (2012) *Individual outcomes: Getting back to what matters*, Edinburgh: Dunedin Academic Press.

Miller, R., Dickinson, H. and Glasby, J. (2011) 'The care trust pilgrims', *Journal of Integrated Care*, vol 19, no 4, pp 14-21.

Mitchell, G.E., O'Leary, R. and Gerard, C. (2015) 'Collaboration and performance: perspectives from public managers and NGO leaders', *Public Performance & Management Review*, vol 38, pp 684-716.

National Evaluation of Sure Start (2002) *Methodology report, executive summary*, London: National Evaluation of Sure Start.

NHS Future Forum (2012) *Integration: A report from the NHS Future Forum*, London: Future Forum.

Nicholas, E., Qureshi, H. and Bamford, C. (2003) *Outcomes into practice: Focusing practice and information on the outcomes people value*, York: York Publishing Services.

Nocon, A. and Qureshi, H. (1996) *Outcomes of community care for users and carers: A social services perspective*, Buckingham: Open University Press.

Nolte, E. and McKee, M. (2008) *Integration and chronic care: A review. Caring for people with chronic conditions: A health systems perspective*, Maidenhead: Open University Press.

ODPM (Office of the Deputy Prime Minister) (2005a) *A process evaluation of the negotiation of pilot local area agreements*, London: ODPM.

ODPM (2005b) *Evaluation of local strategic partnerships: Interim report*, London: ODPM.

ODPM (2007) *Evidence of savings, improved outcomes, and good practice attributed to local area agreements*, London: ODPM.

OECD (Organisation for Economic Co-operation and Development) (1995) *Governance in transition: Public management reforms in OECD countries*, Paris: OECD.

O'Flynn, J. (2009) 'The cult of collaboration in public policy', *Australian Journal of Public Administration*, vol 68, no 1, pp 112-16.

O'Flynn, J. (2014) 'Crossing boundaries: The fundamental questions in public management and policy', in J. O'Flynn D. Blackman and J. Halligan (eds) *Crossing boundaries in public policy and management: The international experience*, London: Routledge, pp 11-44. O'Flynn, J., Buick, F., Blackman, D. and Halligan, J. (2011) 'You win some, you lose some: Experiments with joined-up government', *International Journal of Public Administration*, vol 34, no 4, pp 244-54.

Oliver, C. (1990) 'Determinants of inter-organisational relationships: integration and future direction', *Academy of Management Review*, vol 15, pp 241-65.

Ouwens, M., Wollersheim, H., Hermens, R., Hulscher, M. and Grol, R. (2005) 'Integrated care programmes for chronically ill patients: a review of systematic reviews', *International Journal for Quality in Health Care*, vol 17, pp 141-6.

Øvretveit, J. (1998) *Evaluating health interventions*, Buckingham: Open University Press.

Patton, M.Q. (1997) *Utilization-focused evaluation: The new century text*, London: Sage Publications.

Pawson, R. (2006) *Evidence based policy: A realist perspective*, London: Sage Publications.

Pawson, R. (2013) *The science of evaluation: A realist manifesto*, London: Sage Publications.

Pawson, R. and Tilley, N. (1997) *Realistic evaluation*, London: Sage Publications.

Payne, M. (2000) *Teamwork in multiprofessional care*, Basingstoke: Macmillan.

Peck, E. (2002) 'Integrating health and social care', *Managing Community Care*, vol 10, pp 16-19.

Petch, A., Cook, A., Miller, E., Alexander, H.E., Cooper, A., Hubbard, G. and Morrison, J. (2007) *Users and carer define effective partnerships in health and social care* (http://eresearch.qmu.ac.uk/1258/1/eResearch_1258.pdf).Pfeffer, J. and Salancik, G. (1978) *The external control of organizations: A resource dependence perspective*, New York: Harper & Row.

Phelan, M., Slade, M., Thornicroft, G., Dunn, G., Holloway, F., Wykes, T. et al (1995) 'The Camberwell Assessment of Need: The validity and reliability of an instrument to assess the needs of people with severe mental illness', *The British Journal of Psychiatry*, vol 167, no 5, pp 589-95.

Pierre, J. and Peters, B.G. (2000) *Governance, politics and the state*, New York: St Martin's Press.

Pollitt, C. (1995) 'Justification by works or faith? Evaluating the new public management', *Evaluation*, vol 1, pp 133-54.

Popp, J.K., Milward, H.B., MacKean, G., Casebeer, A. and Lindstrom, R. (2014) *Inter-organizational networks: A review of the literature to inform practice*, Washington, DC: IBM Center for the Business of Government.

Portes, J. (2015) 'A troubling attitude to statistics', Blog post on the National Institute of Economic and Social Research website (www.niesr.ac.uk/blog/troubling-attitude-statistics#.Vqh08IQ2ZX-).

Powell, M. and Dowling, B. (2006) 'New Labour's partnerships: comparing conceptual models with existing forms', *Social Policy and Society*, vol 5, no 2, pp 305-14.

Powell Davies, G., Harris, M., Perkins, D., Roland, M., Williams, A., Larsen, K. et al (2006) *Coordination of care within primary health care and other sectors: A systematic review*, Sydney, NSW: Research Centre for Primary Health Care and Equity, School of Public Health and Community Medicine, UNSW.

Provan, K.G. and Milward, H.B. (1995) 'A preliminary theory of network effectiveness: a comparative study of four community mental health systems', *Administrative Science Quarterly*, vol 40, no 1, pp 1-23.

PSSRU (Personal Social Services Research Unit) (2010) *Adult social care outcomes toolkit*, Canterbury: PSSRU (www.pssru.ac.uk/ascot/).

Punch, K.F. (2014) *Introduction to social research: Quantitative and qualitative approaches* (3rd edn), London: Sage.

Putnam, R. (2003) 'Social capital and institutional success', in E. Ostrom and T.K. Ahn (eds) *Foundations of social capital*, Cheltenham: Edward Elgar Publishing. Qureshi, H., Patmore, C., Nicholas, E. and Bamford, C. (1998) *Outcomes in community care practice: Number five*, York: Social Policy Research Unit.

Raftery, J. (1998) 'Economic evaluation: an introduction', *British Medical Journal*, vol 316, pp 1013-14.

RAND Europe and Ernst & Young (2012) *National evaluation of the Department of Health's Integrated Care Pilots*, Cambridge: RAND Europe.

Robb, B. (1967) *Sans everything: A case to answer*, London: Nelson.

Robson, C. (1993) *Real world research: A resources for real world scientists and practitioner-researchers*, Oxford: Blackwell Publishers.

Rossi, P.H. and Freeman, H.E. (1985) *Evaluation: A systematic approach*, Newbury Park, CA: Sage Publications.

Rowlinson, M. (1997) *Organisations and institutions*, Basingstoke: Macmillan.

Rummery, K. (2009) 'Healthy partnerships, healthy citizens? An international review of partnerships in health and social care and patient/user outcomes', *Social Science & Medicine*, vol 69, pp 1797-804.

Rummery, K. and Glendinning, C. (2000) *Primary care and social services: Developing new partnerships for older people*, Abingdon: Radcliffe Medical Press.

Sackett, D.L., Rosenberg, W.M.C., Gray, J.A.M., Haynes, R.B. and Richardson, W.S. (1996) 'Evidence-based medicine: what it is and what it isn't', *British Medical Journal*, vol 312, pp 71-2.

Schmitt, M.H. (2001) 'Collaboration improves the quality of care: methodological challenges and evidence from US health care research', *Journal of Interprofessional Care*, vol 15, pp 47-66.

Scriven, M. (1991) *Evaluation thesaurus*, Newbury Park, CA: Sage Publications.

Secker, J., Bowers, H., Webb, D. and Llanes, M. (2005) 'Theories of change: what works in improving health in mid-life?', *Health Education Research*, vol 20, pp 392-401.

Shadish, W., Cook, T. and Leviton, L. (1991) *Foundations of programme evaluation: Theories of practice*, London: Sage Publications.

Silverman, D. (2013) *Doing qualitative research: A practical handbook* (4th edn), London: Sage Publishing.

Singleton, R., Straits, B., Straits, M. and McAllister, R. (1988) *Approaches to social research*, Oxford: Oxford University Press.

Smith, P. (1996) *Measuring outcomes in the public sector*, London: Taylor & Francis.

Speak, B.L., Hay, P. and Muncer, S.J. (2015) 'HoNOS – their utility for payment by results in mental health', *International Journal of Health Care Quality Assurance*, vol 28, issue 2, pp 115-28.

Stame, N. (2004) 'Theory-based evaluation and types of complexity', *Evaluation*, vol 10, pp 58-76.

Stoker, G. (1995) 'Regime theory and urban politics', in D. Judge, G. Stoker and H. Wolman (eds) *Theories of urban politics*, London: Sage Publications, pp 54-71. Sullivan, H. (2011) '"Truth" junkies: using evaluation in UK public policy', *Policy & Politics*, vol 39, no 4, pp 499-512.

Sullivan, H. and Skelcher, C. (2002) *Working across boundaries: Collaboration in public services*, Basingstoke: Palgrave.

TaxPayers' Alliance, The (2014) *Bumper book of government waste*, London: The TaxPayers' Alliance.

Thistlethwaite, P. (2011) *Integrating health and social care in Torbay: Improving care for Mrs Smith*, London: The King's Fund.

Thomas, P. and Palfrey, C. (1996) 'Evaluation: stakeholder-focused criteria', *Social Policy and Administration*, vol 30, pp 125-42.

Thompson, G. (1991) 'Comparison between models', in G. Thompson, J. Mitchell, R. Levacic and J. Francis (eds) *Markets, hierarchies and networks: The coordination of social life*, London: Sage Publications.

Thomson, A.M., Perry, J.L. and Miller, T.K. (2009) 'Conceptualizing and measuring collaboration', *Journal of Public Administration Research and Theory*, vol 19, pp 23-56.

Tompkinson, R. (2007) *Shared services in local government*, Aldershot: Gower.

University of East Anglia (2007) *Children's trust pathfinders: Innovative partnerships for improving the well-being of children and young people*, Norwich: University of East Anglia in Association with the National Children's Bureau.

VicHealth (2011) *The partnerships analysis tool*, Melbourne, VIC: Victoria Health Promotion Foundation (www.vichealth.vic.gov.au/~/media/ResourceCentre/PublicationsandResources/General/Partnerships_Analysis_Tool_2011.ashx).

Weinstein, M.C. and Stason, W. (1977) 'Foundations of cost-effectiveness analysis for health and medical practices', *New England Journal of Medicine*, vol 296, pp 716-21.

Weiss, C.H. (1999) 'The interface between evaluation and public policy', *Evaluation*, vol 5, pp 468-86.

Welsh Assembly Government (2011) *Sustainable social services for Wales: A framework for action*, Cardiff: Welsh Assembly Government.

Wiggins, M., Rosato, M., Austerberry, H., Sawtell, M. and Oliver, S. (2005) *Sure Start Plus national evaluation: Final report*, London: University of London.

Williams, I., Robinson, S. and Dickinson, H. (2012) *Rationing in health care: The theory and practice of priority setting*, Bristol: Policy Press.

Williamson, O.E. (1975) *Markets and hierarchies: Analysis and antitrust implications*, New York: Free Press.

Winkworth, G. and Healy, C. (2009) *The Victorian Community Linkages project: Increasing collaboration between State and Commonwealth service systems to improve the safety and wellbeing of vulnerable children in Frankston-Mornington Peninsula and Wodonga*, Canberra, ACT: Institute of Child Protection Studies, Australian Catholic University.

Woodland, R.H. and Hutton, M.S. (2012) 'Evaluating organizational collaborations: Suggested entry points and strategies', *American Journal of Evaluation*, vol 33, no 3, pp 366-83.

Young, A.F. and Chesson, R.A. (2006) 'Stakeholders' views on measuring outcomes for people with learning difficulties', *Health and Social Care in the Community*, vol 14, pp 17-25.

Index

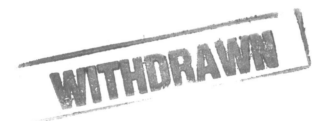